Copyright © by Violeta Bailets

This book is to be used only as a reference and not as medical advice. It is not intended to take the place of medical advice from your physician. You should check with your doctor before beginning any new health regimen or exercise program.

ISBN 978-0-9839973-9-9

Dedicated to my great-grandma, Maria, who was an embodiment of love. To Nina – babuska, my sweet, gentle, caring grandma and most amazing gardener. To mama, Valentina, who taught me creativity, resourcefulness, integrity and strength. Sister, Loreta, a beautiful woman with the ability to deeply listen from the heart and understand. Aunts Lida and Liuda, for showing how to be cheerful and keep faith in every life circumstance.

Focus:

"Teach them to love themselves. Help them feel good in their body. Just as it is..."

~**Swami Ji Balendu**

Contents

ACKNOWLEDGEMENTS   xi

INTRODUCTION
    <u>Personal Story</u>   xii
    <u>Letter from Author</u>   xiii
    <u>4 Principles of Happiness and Health</u>   xiv

Principle 1: BE CALM AND HAPPY FROM YOUR INNER SOURCE   1

  <u>Unlimited Energy And Vitality Chi Gong Routine</u>   2
- Prayer or Focus   2
- Mindful Breathing   2
- Bone Marrow Washing   2
- Standing Tree Meditation   5
- Sending Healing Energy   7
- Thyroid Massage, Scalp Massage and Closing   8

Principle 2: MINDFUL LIVING IN EVERY MOMENT   9

  <u>Mindful Living Tips</u>   10

Principle 3: CONSCIOUS EATING OF LIFE GIVING FOOD FOR VIBRANT ENERGY   16

  <u>Vibrant Health Nutrition Tips</u>   17

Principle 4: PASSION FOR MOVEMENT – FEELING GOOD IN YOUR BODY   25

  Awaken Your Embryonic Fluidity Movement   26
- Cat and Snake Flow   26
- Floating on Your Back   27
- Crawling   29
- Walk on Hands and Knees   30
- Lower and Rise   31
- Dance, Dance, Dance!   32

Feel the Smile in Your Heart – Yoga-and-Pilates Program   34

    <u>Why Yoga and Pilates?</u>   34

    Neck Release   36
- Neck Circles   36
- Neck Extensors   37
- Neck Flexors   38
- Neck Lateral Flexors   39
- Neck Flexor Oblique Stretch   40
- Meditation   41
- Shoulder and Upper Back Release   42
- Seated Spine Lengthener   42
- Cat and Cow   46
- Child's Pose   47
- Downward Facing Dog   48
- Upward Facing Dog to Downward Facing Dog   51
- Kneeling Lunge   52
- Push-ups   54
- Mountain Pose   57
- Shoulder Rotations   58
- Balance to Chair Pose   59
- Warrior I to Proud Warrior to Triangle to Side Angle Bend   60
- Tree Pose   65
- High Lunge to Crescent Moon Lunge to Lunge with Twist   67
- Garland Pose and Peasant's Squat   70
- Boat   72
- Bicycle   75
- Bridge   77
- Side Leg Lifts and Inner Thigh Lifts   79
- Swimming   81
- Locust   83
- Hip Opener   84
- Plow and Shoulder Stand   85
- Legs-up-the Wall   87
- Cobra   88
- Hip Twist   89
- Savasana or Restorative Relaxation   91

<u>Feeling Good in your Body Tips</u>   93

CONCLUSION   101

Bibliography   102

About Author   104

Special Offer   104

ACKNOWLEDGMENTS

Thank you to all of my students, for teaching me with your presence, inquiry, laughter and gentle guidance. Many thanks to my long time students. Too many to name. I have written your names in my heart. Ann, Kathy, Betty, Jane, JoAnna, Suzi, Lorna, Less, Marilyn, Yvonne, Stephanie, Jeanette, Emily, Denise, Linda, Cece, Peggy, Megan, Dana, Ellie, Cheryl, Joan, Jean, Caroline, Betty, Louis, Connie, Gladys, David, Karen and Pat, Pat and Andi, Elaine, JoAnn, Mary, Suzanne, Sue, Charlz and Brenda, Dan, May, Brook, Jan, Sam, Marilyn, Lucinda, Margaret, Toni, Pam, Mary, Chuck, Karen, Fran, April, Julie, Rose, Melody, Marissa, Rosie, Val, Nancy, Pratiti, Kristina, Carol and Lisa.

Jan Rianda for being so giving and tirelessly enthusiastic, while proof reading and helping me to share my message.

Sue Brantley, for teaching me and giving me an opportunity to deepen my understanding and teaching skills for the art and discipline of yoga and Pilates.

My very special friend and naturopathic doctor, Jeannette Lloyns, for nutritional expertise and healing water therapy techniques. You make radiant health possible!

Mark, friend, husband, lover and business partner for your patience and many hours of reading, editing, taking photographs and encouraging me to write. Our beautiful love and life together is a source of my inspiration.

INTRODUCTION

Personal Story

My great-grandmother and grandmother would tell me their life stories and I would love listening to their wisdom about the times long forgotten. What stands out the most is how they were able to find enthusiasm and desire for life in the most difficult times during the World War II and post-war era. Their wisdom imparts to me that happiness lies in the faith that goodness prevails and in the way we relate to ourselves and other people from our hearts with kindness and grace.

My grandmother often used to tell me that health is very important. You can earn a living, you can contribute to society but first you have to take care of your own health. When you have health you can more joyfully and more energetically contribute to the world around you. Ironically, though true, members of my family often sacrificed greatly for others at the price of their own health. My great-grandmother would walk tens of miles at a stretch through the thick Russian forests, which were heavily populated with wolves and sometimes she would have to cross the clumpy bogs in the midst of unknown danger of war to see my great-grandfather to bring him food. On one such occasion, broken by the news of his heroic death and walking many miles through cold and rain, at the age of thirty-five, she damaged her health and was confined to her room for life. Her kind smile, thankfulness and sincerity in prayer kept her living and gracing our family until she was eighty-three. Indeed, our inner contentment and connection to other people is paramount to our health and happiness.

My introspective nature has always led me to puzzle such questions as what is this life about and what is its meaning. I believe that all the things we do are for one purpose – happiness. Even our poor choices reflect our wish to attain happiness in life. My alcoholic father searched for his happiness in the bottle, my great-great-great-grandfather (who was a count of Russia) lost all his estate in gambling, I am sure he was searching for his happiness as well. I myself struggled with an eating disorder while finding my way through struggles in making dietary lifestyle changes.

The writing of this book has been the culmination of a life long learning process of self-test and observation that still continues to this day. I believe the path of learning and self-discovery is never ending. Often the ideas would come after taking an early morning walk with my husband in the woods. During each walk we would embrace each other in our special place among the trees in the quite of the sunrise. Feeling calmness settle in our body and heart. When we are in tune with our hearts, we can discover for ourselves what brings true joy and meanings to life.

"Love bears all things, believes all things, hopes all things, endures all things."

~ Corinthians 13:7-8

Letter from the Author

Lasting health and happiness can only come from within you. The wise old Native American grandfather is telling his grandson the story of two wolves. One wolf is kind, loving, peaceful, giving, thankful and happy, while the other is angry, violent, greedy, resenting and envious. These wolves are having a terrible fight. While listening to the story, the grandson wants to know, "grandfather, which wolf will win"? The grandfather answered, "the one you feed"!

Metaphorically speaking, food is your thoughts and the power they carry when you make your every choice. Every moment of your life you have a choice to be happy or sad, to say a kind word or an angry word, to think positive thoughts or get depressed, to watch TV or read a book, to sit at the concert or dance with joy, to eat fruit or donut. Believe within your whole body, mind and heart that you hold a very special key to health and happiness in your life.

You can become happier and healthier, when you approach life through training of your thinking, body awareness and intelligence of your heart/emotions. I will teach you how you can embrace this power and train your mind, body and heart. These proven techniques are so powerful yet simple that you will instantly feel their benefits. Of course, there are things that will be required on your part such as determination, commitment and practice in thought and action. If you have just started playing a piano, you won't expect yourself to play Beethoven symphony number 9 over night. It takes practice, practice and more practice! It's the same with learning about body awareness, toning your muscles, learning how to think creatively, getting into the habit of making healthy foods choices or opening your heart to love and compassion.

So, do you really want to become healthier and happier? Are you willing to do the work? Do you think about what happiness means to you? Do you plan your healthy meals with enthusiasm? Do you exercise daily and take a great enjoyment in it? I hope you do or will learn how to embrace the PASSION for a lifestyle of health and happiness over time.

It is very important that you learn to live this very moment with radiance of happiness, health, kindness, love, thankfulness and forgiveness in your heart and you shall feel better RIGHT NOW. The secret is to radiate these feelings of inner contentment for what you do in life at this moment, then everything else will come to you in its own time by virtue of your patience.

In peace, joy, love and health,

Violeta Bailets

The Heart's Way 4 Principles of Happiness and Health

- Be calm and happy from your inner source
- Mindful living in every moment
- Conscious eating of life giving food for vibrant energy
- Passion for movement – Feeling good in your body

The first principle is how to BE CALM AND HAPPY FROM YOUR INNER SOURCE. Have you stood by the ocean listening to the ocean waves and feeling wonderful calm within you? Or maybe, you were silently walking through the rye fields and listening to the insects. Whatever it was, I hope you have had one of those moments, when it brings to you a tremendous sense of peace. What if we could cultivate the same inner listening silence and beauty within us and take it wherever we go: to work, to the busy streets, to home? You can, when you realize that the sacred universe starts at your feet, wherever you stand and in every step you take. In this section you will learn meditative Chi Gong techniques that remove blockages and imbalances in your body and mind as it teaches you how to be present in the moment with an open heart, intuitive listening and honesty to oneself.

The second principal, MINDFUL LIVING IN EVERY MOMENT, teaches you to love and accept yourself, grow in wisdom every day by creating daily habits that lead to health and happiness.

The third principal emphasizes that food is your fuel. You won't put rocks into your car's fuel tank, same with your body, the appropriate fuel must be chosen. When you eat wholesome foods, it creates balance in your system which stimulates upbeat thinking, happy mood and vibrant health. CONSCIOUS EATING OF LIFE GIVING FOOD FOR VIBRANT ENERGY is not very difficult. It is actually very cost effective yet requires effort, planning and mindfulness on your part.

The fourth principal is PASSION FOR MOVEMENT – FEELING GOOD IN YOUR BODY. Vibrant and life long health is not about what gadget or equipment you have. Health is not even about working out very hard and doing extreme yoga poses or extreme sports. If you carefully observe nature, you will learn that nothing in nature is in straight lines. Nature is soft, it curves, it gives, it surrounds, it blends, it raises and it falls. We need daily, intelligent movement that moves us from within and teaches how to reclaim natures' way of moving the whole body in a three-dimensional way.

I teach moving body in two ways:

Way #1) non-linear, intuitive as nature has intended. It invites you to move like a child: flowing, shaking, wiggling, turning and moving from instinct and not from the head. It invites you to listen to your body and move in a comfortable, fun and pleasurable ways.

Naturally, your spine becomes more supple, joints more flexible, the movements stimulates lymph system which protects body from harmful pathogens and releases hormones that give a sense of happiness and wellbeing.

Way #2) the second way of moving is based on yoga and Pilates and is presented in a more structured way. Yoga and Pilates help to retrain the habitual movement patterns and strengthen the muscles that otherwise might be underused. So, many times I've heard my students say, "I wish I had started doing yoga earlier in my life or my doctor had told me to do yoga, when everything else has failed". It is never too late to start now. With this book you will learn how to use your own body anytime or anywhere to tone the musculature of your arms and legs, streamline your figure and strengthen your core: abdominal muscles, lower back, hips and buttocks. A strong core means good posture, lower back pain prevention and efficient body function.

It is very important to take care of your body and strive to live without disease; however, living your life, cherishing every day as a miracle, living with zest and laughter are more important than any physical attribute you may have. Building relationships, realizing life is more about love, joy and friendship (less about things and achievements) brings us the only real and lasting happiness, which will be reflected in the sparkle of your eyes!

Principle 1:
BE CALM AND HAPPY FROM YOUR INNER SOURCE

"When the heart is at ease, the body is healthy."
~ Chinese proverb

Your body, mind and emotions are energetically interrelated. By paying attention to your feelings and emotions, and how their effects are manifesting in your body and heart and by practicing breathing and relaxation techniques, you can let go of physical tension, harmonize heart rhythm, while the mind opens up to more creative and intelligent thinking.

The following routine comes from the ancient discipline of Chi Gong. Chi means "life force or energy" and Gong means "flow." Phyllis A. Balch, CNC writes, "[a]ccording to traditional Chinese medicine, this type of exercise wards off illness. It has been linked to reduced blood pressure and increased levels of endorphins, natural body chemicals that relieve pain and maintain mental health." This practice gets you out of your head and teaches you how to listen and speak from the inner silence. It keeps your mind focused in the present moment as you allow yourself to feel the healing energy from the universe to move through your chakras, energy channels in your body, and heal body, mind and soul of physical and emotional stress.

As you do Chi Gong, try to let go of any control. It is up to the energy; it has intelligence and it will move where it is most necessary. By letting go of control, you will notice that with practice you are becoming more spontaneous in your loving speech and action. The joy and laughter will bubble out gently and naturally. Your unique disposition will be welcomed by others in your daily life and your intuitive wisdom will begin to awaken as you receive hints and messages on what is best for you and others at the appropriate times.

<u>Unlimited Energy and Vitality Chi Gong</u> routine includes, *Focus or Prayer* to set your heart and mind on the right track and give yourself a sense of purpose. *Mindfulness Meditation* calms you and can be done by itself at any time of the day. *Bone Marrow Washing* teaches how to let go of unnecessary tension in your body and mind. *Standing Tree Meditation*, focuses on feeling life force moving through you, while renewing and revitalizing your energy levels. And *Sending Healing Energy*, brings to your awareness the most powerful healing tool available to you – healing touch. There is a healing energy in touch like a crying child responds to gentle care even before his physical need has been met. Children and animals are sensitive to healing and loving touch. You can be like a healing mother or father and use gentle, caring and compassionate touch to bring harmony to yourself and others.

To get most of the Meditation and Chi Gong, practice the technique of your choice 1-3 times a day for 5 minutes to 1 hour anytime and anywhere. It is a beautiful experience when you practice Chi Gong outdoors in the fresh air gathering in beauty and peace of nature. Meditation and Chi Gong also can be incorporated into yoga routine or after taking a walk. If you practice for a short period of time, then perform one of the outlined techniques. If you practice for at least 45 minutes than you can comfortably include all of the techniques.

Unlimited Energy And Vitality Chi Gong Routine

- ♦ Prayer or Focus

Begin by setting the intent for your Chi Gong practice. Your focus can be "I am love and compassion," "I am thankful for my health," "Every cell of my body is healthy and happy." Or you can memorize a prayer or a poem that speaks to your heart but most importantly learn to speak from the depths of your soul, honestly, simply and in your own words.

"For the things that you need, you will find, if only you will follow your heart."
~ Stephen Harrod Buhner

- ♦ Mindful Breathing

Purpose: Teaches you how to steady your breath and calm your heart. Awakens inner joy and sense of peace.

Sequence:
1. Sit comfortably in a chair with your feet grounded flat on the floor and spine erect. Rest your arms in your lap with the palms turned up. Relax your shoulders and face. Eyes are gently closed and relaxed. Try to keep your body and eyes very calm and still.
2. Deeply exhale and inhale a few times. Become aware of your breathing. Breathe in very slowly through 4-12 count, hold the breath for the same count you inhaled for, exhale for the same slow count and hold again for the same count that is comfortable for you.
3. Be focused on the way the breath feels, how and where it moves, feel the relaxation it brings to you. If your mind gets distracted, lovingly guide your attention back to your breathing.
4. Practice <u>Mindfulness Meditation</u> for as long as you like.

- ♦ Bone Marrow Washing

Purpose: Improves spine flexibility and releases the toxins from your system. Centers your mind and brightens your attitude.

Sequence:
1. Stand with feet hip distance apart or a little wider, slightly bend your knees, keep lower back neutral. Arms loosely resting at the sides, shoulders relaxed. Eyes are calmly gazing ahead on the ground. Create an inner smile in your heart. You can cultivate an inner smile for a few moments by thinking of something or someone that makes your heart smile. Feel the smile rising deeply from the lower part of your spine and lower abdomen, rising upward through your chest and radiating in your heart.
2. Now focus your attention on your breathing. Let your mind become like a still lake on a beautiful sunny day. If you get distracted, lovingly guide your attention back to your breathing.
3. Rub your palms briskly together to generate heat in your hands.

4. Look upwards and bring your arms out to the sides, turn your palms out and up, inhale and lift the arms upward through your sides above your head. You are gathering a universal energy or chi. You might feel a pleasant sensation, tickling or warmth in the centers of your palms. That's a good indication the chi is moving through your body. Even if you do not feel the chi, it is still moving through you.

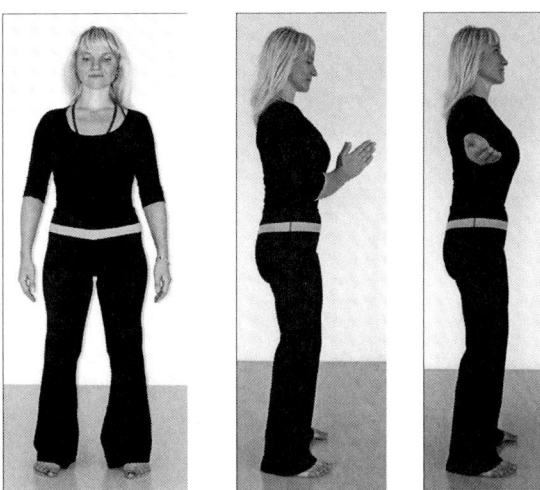

5. As your hands are above your head, turn your palms to face the front part of your skull. Let the energy that you gathered in your palms enter through the crown of your head and into the body. Exhale, direct your gaze inwardly as you very slowly lower your arms downward in front of your body. Feel that you are cleansing the bones of your face, neck, spine and pelvis. When hands reach the level of hips, bend at your hips to cleanse your legs and shins. Go down only as far as your lower back is comfortable; make sure to keep your knees slightly bent. Once you are at your lowest point, turn your palms to face the ground and feel that you are blessing the earth and earth is blessing you. The earth will take all the stagnant and negative energy to be re-circulated and recharged.

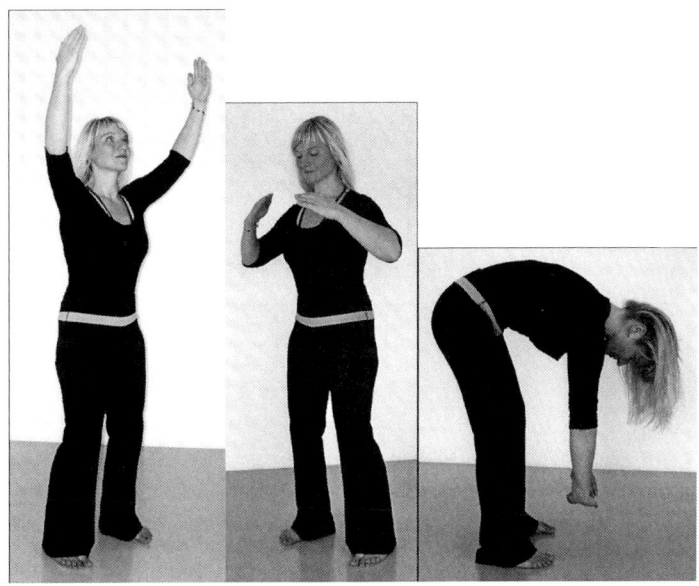

Awareness: *If you keep your elbows slightly bent, does that relax your shoulders? Does keeping connection to the ground through your whole foot make you more stable? Keep knees slightly bent. Now try straightening your knees? Do you feel the difference in your hips or lower back?*

5. Keep feeling a connection to the earth through the soles of the feet and the energy that is being exchanged, inhale and slowly come up vertebra by vertebra to a full upright position with your hands facing lower abdomen. Pause here and breathe for a few cycles. On the inhale, feel how your abdomen, lower back and pelvic floor gently expand. On the exhale, feel how your abdomen and lower back and pelvic floor come in toward each other at your core. Let the breathing pattern be subtle, barely visible, unhurried and at ease.

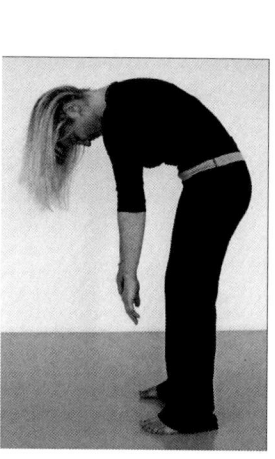
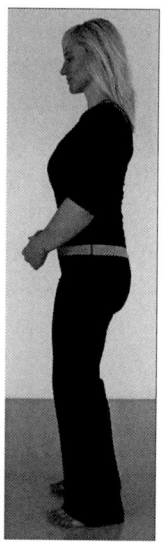

6. Gather chi again, point 4, and repeat 4-9 times.

7. When you are finished, lower your arms down at the sides and focus on what you feel.

Modification:
Perform Bone Marrow Washing without bending forward at your hips. Stay upright and use only arm motion to move the chi in your body.

♦ <u>Standing Tree Meditation</u>

Purpose: Renews and replenishes your energy and vitality, awakens your intuition.

Sequence:

1. Stand with feet hip distance apart or a little wider. Arms loosely resting at your sides, shoulders relaxed. Eyes are calmly gazing ahead on the ground. Create an inner smile in your heart.

2. Turn your palms to the back wall and like a sleep walker raise your arms, leading with the back of your hands and keeping shoulders very relaxed. At about chest level, let your palms face your heart center, mid-chest. Elbows hanging down, shoulders relaxed. Feel that you are radiating the sun from the center of your chest to the world.

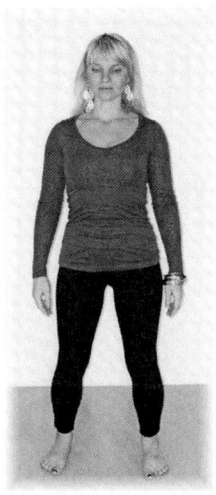 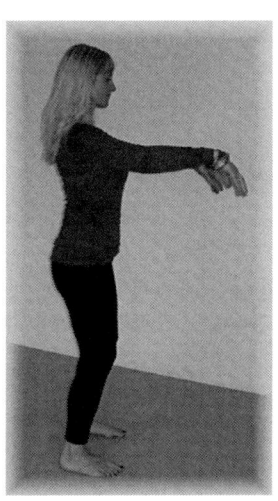 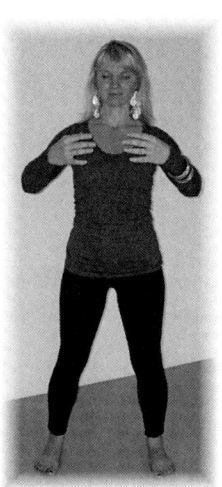

3. Feel 5 points on your body, so-called five-pointed star; soles of your feet, centers of your palms and crown of your head. Now focus on your breathing. As you inhale, draw the energy up through your five points and your skeletal structure into your lower abdomen; on the exhale, send the energy outward to your five points and to all your skin and beyond. Feel how your aura expands. As you exhale, your abdomen, lower back and pelvic floor pull in toward each other. On the inhale, feel that you are gently expanding your abdomen, lower back and pelvic floor. The breathing is very slow and effortless, very quite and barely visible. Breathe for as little as 3 minutes or for as long as 45 minutes.

4. Effortlessly lower your arms slowly down to rest at your sides.

Awareness: *Can you consciously relax shoulders and neck? Imagine the crown of your head is floating upwards. Keep your mind very quiet and focused on your breathing. Let your mind be like a transparent clear lake on a very calm day. Any time your mind wanders to thinking, bring it back to your breathing, energy and sensations.*

Modifications:

1. Your arms can be lower, facing your lower abdomen instead of the chest.

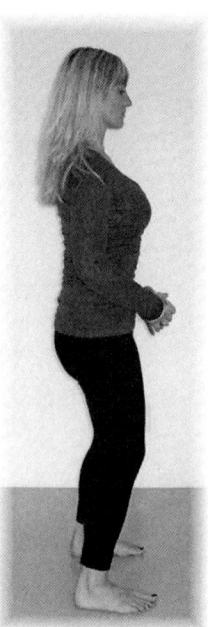

2. You can also turn your palms to the sky or to the earth and feel that you are gathering the chi from heaven or earth.

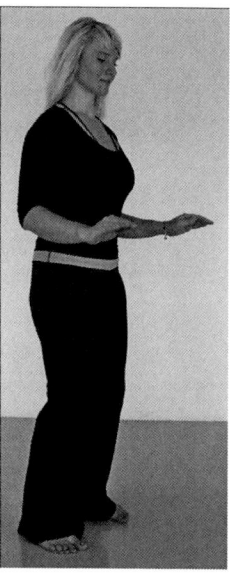

3. You can sit in a chair. If you are seated, rest your hands on your upper thighs with palms facing up. Close your eyes, relax your eyes or gently turn your gaze upwards at the point between the eyebrows. Keep your body and eyes very still and calm.

♦ <u>Sending Healing Energy</u>

Purpose: Healing yourself and others.

Sequence:
1. From the standing tree meditation, light as a feather, lower your arms down by your sides. Focus on your breathing and calmness of mind.

2. Rub your palms vigorously together. Place your hands anywhere on your body you feel you need healing. Scan your body from head to toes. The energy may be needed in your chakras, organs, muscles or joints. Where your hands have the strongest sensation, such as pulsing or warmth, it is an indication where your body calls for energy balance. Place your hands on your body, or barely hover your hands above the area you are healing. Feel how you are sending energy from the universe through your hands. Send healing for a few seconds to 10 minutes, before you move on to another area.

<u>Examples:</u> Back of the neck, solar plexus chakra, tailbone and knees.

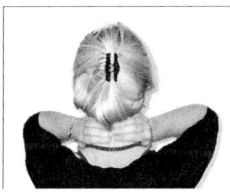 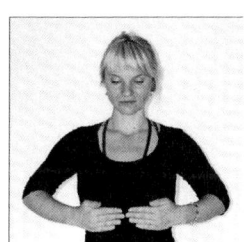 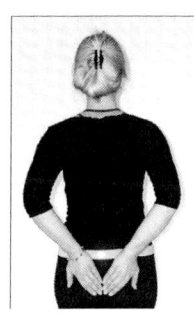 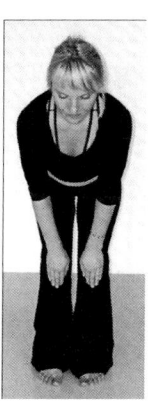

3. Sending Healing Energy to others. Rub your palms, extend arms to the front at about forehead level with elbows bent, shoulders relaxed and palms facing the world. Feel how you are sending healing energy through your palms to someone you know or to whomever needs it.

♦ <u>Thyroid Massage, Scalp Massage and Closing</u>

Purpose: Brings your senses back into the world.

Sequence:

1. Thyroid Massage. Gently and lightly tap right side of the neck, just to the side of the Adam's apple, with your left hand. This stimulates the thyroid gland. Your thyroid gland plays a major role in metabolism and weight control, releases hormones and makes the skin glow. Repeat on the other side.

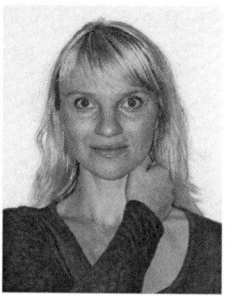

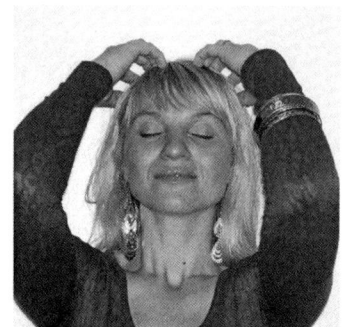

2. Using all ten finger pads in a circular motion, massage all over the scalp for 1 minute. You can also massage your feet or do some gentle yoga stretches.

3. Place one hand on your heart. Place the other hand on your lower abdomen and pause for a few moments. Feel peace and calmness radiating through your being. You can say a prayer or affirmation. Feel it with your whole being – your thoughts of peace and goodwill manifesting.

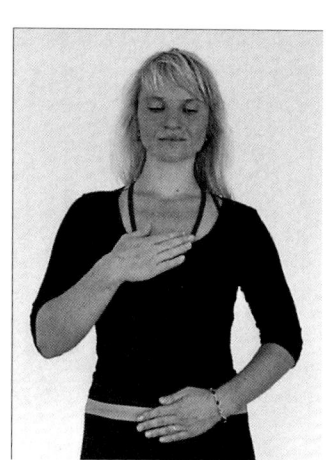

Principle 2:
MINDFUL LIVING IN EVERY MOMENT

Our life is about choices we make on a moment-to-moment basis. Every choice we make carries its own consequences. In the development of wisdom, one needs to slow down, listen to ones intuition (heart) and then take the time to evaluate the choices more carefully. Ask yourself a question: does this really lead me to the true source of happiness or is it only a temporary gratification of my immediate desires?

Every cell in our body has memory. Our cells are intelligent. We can train ourselves to be healthy or unhealthy, happy or unhappy, joyful or sad. The repeated actions and thoughts become our habits. For instance if you allow anger to manifest into your life repeatedly, then that's what kind of memory you are wiring into the structure of your cells in your whole body. And when a critical situation arises, your impulse will be to become angry. Or one might drink just one small alcoholic beverage often enough for it to become a desire to drink every night. Later it becomes necessary to boost your mood with alcohol, which fosters addiction. Compound actions, behaviors, repetitive thought and emotional patterns are the building blocks of who we become in the process.

You can retrain and rewire your cells by first noticing why you do what you do and how it makes you feel. Meditation, Chi Gong, introspection, self-analysis and observation are tools you can use to develop the habits you want. So, instead of getting angry, stop, sit down, consciously slow down, set everything aside, perform Chi Gong meditation technique and then ask yourself the question, why am I acting from impulse. What am I thinking? What I am saying to myself? Where is the missing link between my emotions and behavior? Try going in the opposite direction of your impulse. Pause in silence and take a long walk. The more often you replace your impulses that lead you to unhappiness with thoughts, self-encouragement and actions that promote inner peace and love, the more you will be acting from conscious wisdom that leads to growth and discovery of endless creative solutions!

When you read <u>Practical Mindful Living Tips</u>, keep in mind that sometimes it takes time to rewire your cells and change your habits, your ways and your attitudes. The first step is to acknowledge which area of life or your attitude you would like to improve or develop. Evaluate the intensity of your desire for change. As Kevin Trudeau, the author of <u>How to Manifest your Desires,</u> teaches how to determine if you are ready to make changes in your life. Ask yourself, how strongly do I want to wake up every morning and feel wonderful? Ask yourself such a question for any desire you have in your life and then rate the intensity of your desire on the scale of 1-10. If your desire is between 8 and 10, and if you are willing to make sacrifices, then you are on the right track. For example, you are overweight and would like to loose weight. Are you willing to give up eating after 7pm? Are you willing after work instead of watching TV to take an exercise class? Are you willing to do what it takes and do it with great enthusiasm? Of course, there will be times when you will stumble and "even fall", but you are willing to take the steps, sometimes forward, sometimes backward. The only wrong thing you can do is not to keep on trying! The more you repeat something over and over, the easier it gets for you to live it.

"The difference between the top performers and average or mediocre performers in not a huge difference in talent or ability. Often, it is just a few small things done consistently and well, over and over again."
~Brian Tracy

Mindful Living Tips

- **Live by 5 Reiki principles**

    You have a right to experience any feelings. Yet holding onto the emotions can result in physical and emotional pain. Acknowledge your emotions and then try to move on.

    <u>I won't get angry today</u> [anger blinds us and we may act irrationally, bringing harm to ourselves and others. It is OK to disagree and act upon your convictions, but act from a place of calmness and respect. Learn to communicate your emotions with clarity and compassion toward the listener. The ability to be kind, true and honest to yourself and others leads to wisdom in your speech and choices. If you find yourself getting angry, try to walk out of the room and perform Mindful Breathing as described on p. 10. When our breath is calm and even; then we can discuss the matter more peacefully. Thich Nhat Hanh teaches visualization technique how to let go of anger: visualize you and the person who made you angry 200 years from now, it puts everything in a different perspective.]

    <u>I won't worry today</u> [life can sometimes get difficult and when we don't have control of the circumstances, we worry. Yet worry doesn't made things better. Worry is associated with fear and uncertainty. As Franklin D. Roosevelt said, "all we have to fear is fear itself." Try to find the source of your fear and face it, acknowledge it and plan your pro-active methods in empowering yourself and finding ways to replace your fear with wisdom, action, humor, laughter and faith.]

    <u>I will work honestly today</u> [practice meditative daily activity, do all things with mindfulness and care. Listen to the honesty of your heart (does this really lead me to the source of happiness) as you make decisions about the choices you make in your life.]

    <u>I will express gratitude today</u> [practice contentment and cherish simplicity in life. Walk outside, rain or shine, and learn to see beauty and joy everyday in your life. Realize that happiness, humility and contentment have to be learned anew every day. Be present: enjoy the flower, the winter's cold, the summer's breeze… This life is too short to be in a hurry! If you are not here and not in the moment, then how can you truly enjoy life, listen attentively and give your infinite joy and love to yourself and others?]

    <u>I will honor every living being</u> [respect elders and your parents for they have given you life and hopefully raised you with love and care. When you communicate with another human being, give your full attention, listen with an open heart, relax your shoulders and lift your heart center, be absorbed in the

moment and radiate the willingness to connect by listening and communicating from your heart center. Also honor earth by living in harmony with nature and leaving this earth a green and healthy place to live for generations to come.]

- ♦ **Reduce stress in your life.**

The antidote for stress in your life is living your life with enthusiasm. "Enthusiasm" from Greek means "with God." Live your life with purpose, love and contentment. Recognize that every life experience you've had along your way, no matter how painful it might have been, has led you to the present moment. Your life is your learning experience, and you have the power to make the "now" more meaningful and richer based on your past.

"Happiness is like a butterfly. The more you chase it, the more it eludes you. But if you turn your attention to other things, it comes and sits softly on your shoulder."
~ Henry David Thoreau

"The greatest happiness of life is the conviction that we are loved – loved for ourselves, or rather loved in spite of ourselves.
~ Victor Marie Hugo

- ♦ **Finish your goals.**

Unfinished tasks and projects zap your energy. So look around and make a plan today how you are going to complete something that you really wanted to do, yet it never gets finished. By completing a task you will boost your energy levels, self-confidence and enthusiasm.

> *Boost your enthusiasm for the difficult task by first completing something that comes to you naturally yet it is still challenging. Pay attention to the kind of effort and self-encouragement it takes for you to finish what you've started. Also, it is very exciting and exhilarating to know you have done something worthwhile. Take the feelings and emotions that you experienced in the process of completing the task that came to you naturally and remind yourself of these feelings when you are doing something that is less enjoyable or more difficult for you.*
>
> *If you are happy and excited when you are reaching for your goal, then you are already living your dream. Being happy now is the key to life. When and how you reach your goal no longer matters. It will come to you in time, if you have passion for what you do. Radiate the happiness of your heart and soul right now. Take the time to make your journey special, beautiful and enjoy every step along the way, so when you reach your destination you will not feel empty or exhausted.*

- **Stay away from smoke and smoking.**

    No need to say much about smoking, as we all know how bad it is for us. Simply quit… You are devastating yourself. Find your way, try again and again and never give up until you have quit, no matter how long it takes! It is very helpful to meet with people who have reached their goals; look for inspiration and follow their example.

    > *This can help not only for smoking, but for anything else you really want to overcome in your life. Replace your harmful habit with something constructive. That way you are not just saying "no" to your habit, as it might only intensify the need and make it difficult for you to change. Instead find something that you really want in your life, and build it into your life by replacing a harmful habit with a self-enriching habit. For example, you love gardening but you want to quit smoking. Plant a garden, learn how to grow peppermint and drink peppermint tea or go to your garden every time you crave a cigarette! It takes time to change; don't give up and keep trying. Every failure gets you closer to your goal! Keep on trying until you succeed!*

- **Simplify and organize.**

    Live in a place that is clean, light, airy and uncluttered to open up your thinking and creativity. Recycle and give some things away to a local charity organization to make your home more organized. When we live simply, we also improve our enjoyment for life and health.

- **Put your favorite clothes on.**

    If you wait for a special occasion, it might never come. It doesn't matter if it's Monday or Friday, every day is a miracle, so celebrate it. If you feel like wearing something special and colorful, go ahead. Celebrate and share the light!

- **Connect to your roots.**

    On the other side of the spectrum, sometimes allow yourself to just be. Try not to worry about your nails, hair, clothing – get outside into the wilderness, play in the dirt, connect with the earth, run on the beach barefoot, pick berries and sow seeds in the soil.

- **Watch less TV and do something that stimulates you, something that you truly enjoy.**

It is OK to watch movies once in a while but reading a book or learning something really well is so much better. Reading will open up new neuron pathways in your brain. As Steve Chandler said, "on which side of the screen do you want to live? When you watch TV, you are living someone else's life and paying for it." Often by watching TV or seeking constant entertainment, we hide and suppress our true inner feelings, emotions and yearnings. So, why won't you live your own life in the way you always dreamed of doing. Introspect your potential and choose activities that stimulate your growth, skill and mastery.

- **Live with a sense of community.**

Health in the Native American tradition is defined by "we are all related." If you have a strong and beautiful inner foundation and build a community of people whom you can trust whole-heartedly and in return be trusted, then your life will have meaning.

In the book Outliers Malcolm Gladwell tells a story. In the 1950s, when heart disease was on the rise in the United States, there was a community of Italians, Rosetans, living in the hills of Pennsylvania. Their death rate from heart disease was 50 percent lower compared to the overall United States. All other disease causing deaths where lower by 30 percent. Scholars investigating their diet were surprised to find a diet containing plenty of fat and sweets. On top of that they didn't exercise. Next, they examined their heritage, and they found that their ancestors had heart troubles and their death rate was higher. Could it have been their location with fresh mountain air as the source of their health? No, because the neighboring communities didn't enjoy the same good health. Finally, they looked into their lifestyle and found that they took time to visit and helped one another, the grandparents were living among their grandchildren, and the elders were respected and included in the life of the family. This sense of connection to one another was the source of their wellbeing.

- **Give and receive hugs daily.**

Gentle touch is one of the most important expressions of love, compassion, healing and friendship. Holding someone and allowing yourself to be held, can convey your love more than any words can express. "Four hugs a day will help you survive the blues," says social scientist Dr. Virginia Satir, "but a dozen are better. Our pores are places for messages of love. Being able to have physical contact is very important."

- **Laughter does miracles for your health and soul.**

Smiling, laughing, having fun is our birthright. Look at the babies and children; they are the masters of bringing joy into life. Even laughing for no reason is better than not laughing at all. Improve your health and mood with daily laughing!

- **Love yourself.**

    Awareness: Stand in front of the mirror. What do you see? What thoughts come to you as you see your own reflection?

    Awareness: Stand in front of the mirror. Look with a quite mind, send yourself a gift of love and acceptance from the depths of your heart. Take a few very deep breaths. How does this make you feel?

    Awareness: As you face someone can you see the reflection of yourself? Can you understand the same basic human need to love and to be happy? Can you "see" the heart? Can you connect with the soul? What if you would be blind, what matters then?

    I never think of my age, never – I could be 20 or 100. I never think about it, I'm just me."
    ~ Jack Lalanne

- **Finish your day calmly.**

    One hour before sleep, take time to unwind. Make your sleeping environment cozy and conducive to rest: dim lights, play soft music, light candles etc. Sip calming tea, read inspirational literature and meditate.

    When all is done, can you sleep peacefully like a baby. Learning the ability to calm your thoughts is the magic solution to peaceful sleep. Unless controlled, our thoughts will often run endlessly. In order to keep our mind calm we need to focus on bodily sensations and breathing. This will bring our attention into the present moment and away from restless thoughts.

    Relaxation technique: While performing this technique, keep your mind focused on body sensations, breathing and relaxation. Lay flat on your back. Tense your body one body part at a time and relax: gradually tense left foot for 3 seconds and then gradually completely relax, tense right foot and relax. Keep repeating, contract and release, for the rest of body: left calf, right calf, left thigh, right thigh, left buttock, right buttock, lower abdomen, upper abdomen, left side of chest, right side of chest, left arm and right arm.

    Now relax your body completely, including your face and neck, let go and do breathing awareness exercise. Let your belly rise and fall like an ocean wave with your breathing. Try not to control your breathing. When it comes it comes, when it goes it goes. Imagine the whole universe is breathing through you. Surrender your whole body and being into the peacefulness. You might feel lightness and warmth in your body. Relax and drift to sleep.

- **Sleep restfully.**

    Some people need more sleep, others less. Most of us need 7-9 hours on average. The best time to go to sleep is between 9 and 10 p.m. and wake-up early in the morning. As Kevin Trudeau, the author of <u>Natural Cures</u> states, " [t]he body secrets healing hormones during the times between 10:00 p.m. and 2 a.m.. If you are the person who goes to sleep very, very late, you are not giving your body the proper amount of hours it needs to secrete the hormones that rejuvenate, recharge and refresh your body." The rest is very important for your body to heal and feel at its best during the day!

    Practice restorative sleeping, by sleeping on your back with no pillow or a small pillow under your head. Arms resting at your sides. Or you can place a pillow on your abdomen and place your hands on the pillow, as if hugging it, for the comfort of your shoulders. If you have hip or lower back discomfort place a pillow under your knees to relieve the pressure. It takes time to get used to sleeping in this position without tossing and turning. If you've done yoga, you know this as Savasana pose, which brings the body into healing, balance and rest.

    An alternative way to sleeping would be a fetal position. Lying on your side with knees bent. One pillow between the knees for lower back and hip comfort and another pillow under your head, which brings your neck into alignment with the rest of the spine.

    A habit of sleeping on high pillows or on stomach might be comfortable yet it constricts the neck, shoulders and lungs.

> *Listen to your body rhythms. If you wakeup early and can't go back to sleep, even if it is 2 a.m. in the morning, then get up, meditate, pray, read, write and create. As Wayne Dyer put it, the world is very quite at night and is a good time for cultivating your spiritual awakening.*

Principle 3:
CONSCIOUS EATING OF LIFE GIVING FOOD FOR VIBRANT ENERGY

Why do we eat? We eat to sustain physical life and for pleasure. Sometimes we eat for no good reason: tired, depressed, sad, bored, addictions and desire for very rich, sugary and salty foods. Sometimes we want to please and not to offend someone by eating something that is being offered yet knowing it isn't what is best for our health. Yet truly, the food we eat is the source of how we feel physically, emotionally and even spiritually. The person who is malnourished or who eats junk foods will act restless, unfocused and irritable, while the person who eats a wholesome diet will be able to develop more muscle tone, have strong bones, enjoy a peaceful and happy outlook on life, see and communicate with clarity, have better relationships and learn new skills easier.

The act of eating comes from moment to moment choices. The choices should be based on your mental intelligence on what your body needs: water, carbohydrates, proteins, fiber, good fats, vitamins and minerals. Your emotional intelligence plays a major role in the way you eat: Is this really what I am hungry for? Is this really good for me? Am I present and enjoy every moment when I am eating?

Conscious Eating is a skill that develops overtime, a learning process to experiencing the food beyond the mouth. Pause and feel: is the food you are eating really nourishing every organ in your body or is it only satisfying your sense of taste. We should recognize that food is a gift and a source of keeping your body healthy for a lifetime. We should learn about its source, prepare our own meals often and appreciate every moment of the process of gathering food, preparing it with gratitude and love, and finally savoring the smell, the colors and tasting every bite while being very relaxed physically and emotionally.

When you eat from the place of consciousness, you will notice you body normalizes the weight without following extremely strict diet. When you stop before each meal and open yourself to the true need of the present moment, your digestion and emotional relationship with food will greatly improve.

Awareness: *Next time you want to eat, stop and place your hands on your abdomen. Take a few very deep breaths. Allow yourself to relax, listen to the signals your body sends to you. Breathe for as long as you need to hear the answer on what you really need at this moment. It might not even be food, it might be a need to take a nap and recharge, it might be that you simply need to talk with someone about the day you've had today...*

Awareness: *When you are eating your food, slow down, breathe, and notice, in what physical and emotional state you are in. Open yourself to accepting your food, to accepting your body, feel how by loving yourself for who are, you are able to nourish your body. The body relaxes, shoulders soften, posture lifts to free your abdomen for good digestion. Your meals become an enjoyable and nourishing experience!*

Vibrant Health Nutrition Tips

- **Drink pure water.**

  Because most people do not eat enough vegetables and fruits, the usual recommended water intake is eight 8-10 oz glasses of water per day.

  Often we mistakenly associate hunger for thirst. If you have a tendency to overeat, watch your water intake closely. Make sure to drink sufficient amounts of water and eat fresh produce, include natural food that have high water content such as cucumber and watermelon during the day. You can flavor your water with a squeeze of natural lemon or lime juice. Adjust your water intake during hot weather or when exercising as we sweat more and need to drink more water at these times.

  Water dilutes your digestive juices. So, it is better to drink and eat your meals separately. You can drink 15 minutes before a meal and 1 hour after the meal.

- **Reduce or eliminate alcohol, coffee and caffeinated drinks.**

  One of the worst things you can do to yourself is to drink diet sodas (with artificial cancer causing sweeteners) and sugar loaded soft drinks. Caffeine acts interferes with digestion and calcium assimilation. So, drink coffee in moderation without artificial sweeteners and creamers. Instead add milk and honey or other natural sweetener.

  Alcohol is a depressant and it stimulates gastric acid secretion, which creates too much acid in the stomach making it difficult to have balanced digestion. Drink alcohol in moderation!

- **Drink your water warm or room temperature. Eat your food warm.**

  Two extremes, cold and hot foods and liquids, disturb your internal chi, digestion, and damage your organs. So drink liquids and eat foods that are moderately warm or cool.

  > *When ordering water at the restaurant, always ask, "No ice, please."*

- **Eat breakfast!**

  It does not need to be big, but you should eat something nutritious that has fiber and protein, which keeps you from binge eating later in the day.

- **Make lunch your biggest meal, not dinner.**

You do not need calories while you sleep. Eating a heavy dinner results in unused calories which your body stores as fat. You will sleep much better if you make your dinner light. If you eat breakfast and your lunch, you will experience less hunger at dinner time. It might take some changes in your schedule to make this switch. With a little planning you can make the transition easier.

> *Cook your dinner in the evening but don't eat it until the next day for breakfast or lunch.*
>
> *Ask your boss for a one- hour lunch break, if you only have 30 minutes. It is important to relax as you eat.*
>
> *Bring lots of fresh vegetables with you to work. It takes minimum preparation to eat your vegetables raw. Without any salad dressing or slicing. Just bite and chew!*
>
> *In the evening tonight, instead of watching TV and eating, go for a relaxing walk and then read a book.*

- **Can you afford not to eat organic?**

Organic food is super food! Your body is designed to eat wholesome foods. Our bodies get quality nutrients from natural food sources. Sometimes vitamin and mineral supplements are appropriate, yet nothing will substitute for the nourishment you receive from foods that are as close to their natural state as possible. Eating organic might seem to be more expensive initially, yet pesticides, herbicides and chemical fertilizers eventually take their toll on your health as well as your wallet. How much is your health worth to you?

> *Think: I eat foods that are as close to the raw, organic, natural state as possible.*
>
> *You cannot overeat raw vegetables. "They are full of vital force enhancing vitality." Be creative with your vegetables. Consider eating your garden weeds. You will find that one of the most nutritious vegetables is the common dandelion. Dandelion is a bitter tonic that improves digestion by stimulating kidneys and liver function. However we often shy away from food that tastes bitter. Using a variety of herbs to flavor your food can be fun and exciting. When we learn about culinary herbs and the way nature moves with seasons, then we can learn about the power of healing.*

- **If possible, buy locally grown food.**

Local vegetables are closer to you, which mean's they retain their nutrients in the shipping process. Your meals will be much more satisfying and palatable and you will surely taste the difference! Even better, create a family garden plot so the whole family can get involved in a wholesome outdoor activity. Growing your own organic vegetables is an easy and very satisfying way to provide yourself and your family with the best possible food.

- **Eat variety of foods.**

Experiment with wholesome foods that you normally avoid, such as kohlrabi or shitake mushrooms. Eating a varied diet will ensure the body gets all the nutrients it needs. Avoid food boredom by including foods that are exotic and healthy such as pineapple and guava to keep your senses alive!

- **Eat a healthy diet.**

Contrary to popular belief, eating healthy is very easy. It takes no more time than usual and in the long run is less expensive. How much does it take to wash a fruit or peel a banana - seconds! How much effort does it take to prepare raw vegetables? Just wash and eat. Healthy fruit and vegetable snacks are high in fiber. Fiber will fill you and you will be less hungry and more careful in selecting your food for main meals. A varied diet is vital and necessary to good health.

Carbohydrates are important for energy, proteins for muscle development and good fats for energy. So vary your diet and combine your food groups to make them balanced and nutritious.

Sample Menu and water intake example for optimal weight loss and health:
Early morning: *1-2 cups of water. You can add 1-3 tsp. of apple cider vinegar or freshly squeezed lemon juice, which restores pH levels in your system.*
Breakfast: *Eat a nutritious breakfast! Have something that has plenty of fiber and include protein in your breakfast to give you a good energy boost for the day ahead. Your breakfast can be yogurt with almonds, whole wheat bagel and bananas or eat an omelet with a baked potato, a leftovers from dinner.*
Before lunch: *2-3 cups of water. Remember you can flavor your water with lemon, unsweetened cranberry juice or a tad of honey to make it more palatable.*
Snack: *Apples or freshly made vegetable juice: 6 carrots, ½ beet, small cucumber, 1 stock of celery, 2 handfuls of spinach*.*
Lunch: *Big fresh organic salad with richly colored vegetables with avocado, nuts and seeds. You can also eat a piece of chicken, potatoes and steamed vegetables. For your salad dressing use low sodium options apple cider vinegar, olive oil, and a dash of Bragg's Liquid Aminos*.*
Before dinner: *2-3 cups of water.*
Mid afternoon snack: *raw carrots.*
Skip Dinner or eat very lightly: *Steamed kale with brown rice. Or vegetable soup and raw red bell pepper.*
Optional later in the evening: *Unsweetened herbal tea*.*

*Fresh made vegetable juice is rich in vitamins and it should be consumed within 15 minutes after juicing. It is best to eat your fruits because their juice is very high in sugar.

*Bragg's Liquid Aminos is made from soybeans. It tastes a lot like soy sauce without any additional salt or preservatives added. It contains protein and adds flavor to your food. However, use it very sparingly as it does contain naturally occurring sodium.

*Herbal teas are naturally caffeine free. Peppermint or ginger tea stimulates digestion and soothes upset stomach. Hibiscus has antioxidants. Catnip and chamomile promotes restful sleep. If you are interested in experimenting with soothing herbal tea flavors, there are many other herbs to learn about. The green tea contains caffeine, yet it is also a good source of antioxidant compounds that protect our cells from damaging effects and play an important role in disease prevention. Drinking green tea in the morning or earlier part of the day can be a good addition to your diet.

IMPORTANT: Preparing a shopping list before heading out to the store makes shopping efficient and helps you to stick with your healthy choices.

<u>Sample Shopping List:</u>
Bananas
Organic Apples
Organic Cucumbers
Organic Tomatoes
Organic lettuce
Avocados
Extra virgin olive oil
Lentils
Brown Rice
Raw almonds
Unsulfured dried apricots
Organic Plain Yogurt
Organic Chicken
Curry powder
Garlic

Shopping rule 1: Buy most of your groceries in the living section of the store, where you find fruits and vegetables.

Shopping rule 2: Read food labels before you buy. If you don't understand the ingredient on the package or you need a chemical dictionary to look the ingredient up, then don't buy the product. Or "if your grandma doesn't know what that is, then pass the strange food by." Go back to the basic, wholesome foods!

Awareness: Look around: kitchen, refrigerator, cupboard, office, coffee table. What do you see? Any candy or chocolate? Or is it unsalted raw nuts and rasins? Any white flour bread or cake? Or is it homemade whole grain and seed bread? Throw everything away that isn't healthy and fill your environment with

> *dried fruit, raw nuts and seeds, fresh fruit, vegetables and grains! Please don't give sugary snacks to someone else yet be true to your decision to promote health conscious awareness. If you eliminate from your immediate environment unhealthy foods, then you will be more inclined to eat a wholesome diet! By changing yourself, you will inspire the people around you to evaluate their choices.*

- **Eat your food slowly.**

Sit down to enjoy your meals and try to eat more home-made meals. Enjoy this great life's pleasure; your body will respond with better digestion and nutrient absorption. Say a blessing or invocation before the meal and you will feel more relaxed and thankful for food. Sit for at least 5 minutes after the meal or take a short walk. You should get up from the table satisfied and be comfortable taking a slow walk outdoors without any discomfort after the meal. Did you know that fresh air can actually help you digest your food?

- **Eat only when you are calm.**

Avoid eating food when you are emotionally charged. Also avoid stressful and emotional conversations during the meal. Turn off the TV and instead you can play music. Let your meal be an enjoyable experience!

- **Eat with moderation.**

It is better to eat small meals than one big meal in one sitting. Try to get up from the table before you get that "I am so stuffed" feeling. Ideally, your last meal should be 3 hours before your normal bedtime. If you get hungry in the late evening, eat something that is quickly assimilated, such as some fruit, or herbal drink tea sweetened with honey.

- **What if you splurge.**

Make a commitment to follow healthy dietary habits most of the time. But we all have moments when we want to eat our favorite foods, especially during the holiday season. I suggest that you eat a well-balanced diet and once in a while, allow yourself to splurge and have an occasional treat. If we think that we have to be perfect all the time, we will be setting ourselves for disappointment.

- **Feel energetic.**

Fatigue and tiredness can be a reflection of poor diet and food intolerance. Try to eliminate two main energy zappers from your diet: sugar and white, refined grain and flour products as these slowdown the digestive process. Instead of white sugar, use dried fruit, stevia or sparingly sweeten your food with raw sugar, agave nectar, molasses or honey. Instead of white rice or bleached flour products, eat brown rice, quinoa and other whole grains.

Also, diets high in salt, dairy and highly processed, packaged foods should be avoided. If you suspect food intolerance to dairy, corn, nuts, wheat or soy, then eliminate that item for one month before reintroducing it into your diet. An adverse reaction is proof positive, you have a food related allergy or intolerance. You should have a reaction within one to two hours after eating the food. Delayed signs might also include indigestion or feeling unusually tired or sluggish the next day.

Try a cleansing diet one day a week. Exclude rich foods and alcohol as they can accumulate uric acid and precipitate in the joints of the body over time. Also exclude all animal products. Give your system a break and detoxify. Always start the day by drinking at least 8 oz. of water with 1-3 tsp. of apple cider vinegar or freshly squeezed lemon juice, which restores pH levels in your system. Eat vegetables, especially green leafy vegetables, raw, steamed or sautéed. Eat whole (gluten-free) grains such as quinoa and brown rice. Eat nuts and seeds as a source of your protein and good fat, especially almonds, sunflower and pumpkin seeds. Drink pure water. You can also drink some herbal teas. Eat a little fruit; however, avoid oranges and other sweet citrus fruit as their oils can be hard on our digestive system.

Creative dietary options:

Instead of salt, use kelp granules, which are rich in minerals. Use more herbs to flavor your food.

Instead of sugar, and any other kind of sweetener, especially corn syrup, which I call "sugar on steroids", use natural sweeteners sparingly. Eat a piece of fresh or dried fruit whenever you have a sugar craving.

Instead of red meats, eat chicken and fish in moderation.

Instead of bread and flour products, eat potatoes, brown rice and other whole grains.

Instead of coffee or alcohol, drink herbal teas.

Instead of salad dressings, use extra virgin olive oil or flax seed oil; and apple cider vinegar. Add a little Bragg Liquid Aminos, sprinkle some kelp and herbs. Apple cider vinegar is the only vinegar that is compatible with normal pH levels in our body.

Eat nothing that contains hydrogenated oils or margarine; these clog your arteries. Never heat cooking oils to the point of smoke. Heated oil oxidizes and creates carcinogens, as does barbecued food. Even better yet, do not cook with low temperature oils; instead sauté in water or in the high temperature grape-seed oil.

> Black pepper should be avoided for the most part, as it can irritate the digestive lining. Use plenty of cayenne pepper, ginger and raw pure garlic in your diet, which are wonderful circulatory and digestive system stimulants.

- **Healthy elimination.**

    Digestion = regularity = vibrant health. Intestinal flora plays a major role in our overall health including the proper functioning of the immune system. One reason for difficulty may be the lack of digestive enzymes for a specific food you are eating. You might need to add some enzymes and additional natural fiber to promote regularity, at least 3 times a week.

    Your digestion will significantly improve if you eliminate all flour and sugar products and add plenty of raw vegetables. Eat plain yogurt or take probiotics to improve intestinal flora with beneficial bacteria.

    Never force yourself to eliminate, take the time to spend time on the toilet. Do gentle breathing exercises or perform Kegel exercise as it has been described in the Intelligent Exercise Tips (Strengthen your pelvic floor p. 96). However, instead of holding the contraction for 5 seconds, make one to two second contractions around rectal area, which should stimulate ease of elimination.

- **Eat your vitamins.**

    Get most of your vitamins from food sources.

    Vitamin C is a vital antioxidant, which supports the immune system. Eat raw red bell peppers, broccoli, papaya – foods rich in Vitamin C.

    Eat fish at least once a week or ingest flax seed oil. Fish and flax oils contain Omega-3 fatty acids that keep your heart healthy, improve skin condition and stimulate brain function.

    Sunshine is a good source of Vitamin D. It is also found in fish, milk products and eggs, which promotes healthy bones and boosts immunity.

    Your anti-aging food is dark green leafy vegetables, which are a natural source of vitamins A, C, E, K, folate and minerals calcium, iron, potassium and magnesium. My favorite green super food is common dandelion!

    Keep your bones healthy, prevent heart disease, headaches, constipation, relieve legs cramps, improve circulation and your overall health by eating foods rich in Magnesium (pumpkin seeds, brazil nuts, quinoa, spinach and almonds).

    Proper thyroid function stimulates metabolic rate and energy levels. Get your iodine by seasoning your food with seaweeds such as kelp and dulse.

Cruciferous family plants such as cabbage, broccoli, cauliflower and kale have many healing compounds "that could help reverse and prevent cancers and other aging-related diseases," according to the scientists from the University of Alabama, Birmingham.

Even if we eat a variety of healthy and vitamin rich foods, still today's soil is so diminished in nutrients that many of us lack essential nutrients as a result. That's why I recommend taking at least a good quality multivitamin made from real food. However, we are all different and it is best to consult with a naturopathic physician who can test you to determine which best supplements are for you. I like supplements made from real raw foods. When taking supplements, proper absorption is very vital. Make sure your vitamins and minerals are from natural sources and not chemically produced in the laboratory. Also, if they are in liquid or powder form, they are much easier to assimilate.

Awareness: *Feed your body like a growing plant. With the right nutrient combination, you will notice radiant skin, stronger hair and nails. Try growing a living plant and see what it takes to keep it happy and alive.*

Caution: Always consult your nutritionist when taking supplements. Discuss with your doctor, if you are pregnant or nursing.

Principle 4:
PASSION FOR MOVEMENT – FEELING GOOD IN YOUR BODY

We came from water, and we are mostly fluids: water, blood, lymph, cerebral spinal fluid, fat. That is one of the reasons that drinking pure water is so important for us! Our body is like a river: when we move fluidly, we are awakening the state when we felt safe and secure in our mother's womb. When our movements are fluid and harmonized, we are well. When we become too rigid and inflexible, we are losing the natural ability to be healthy. When you move fluidly, you are in your own rhythm, you move in accord with your own body as nature has designed you to move. Paying attention to what is comfortable, pleasurable and healing to you is your innate body's wisdom you must cultivate!

Consider this from Andrew Weil's book Spontaneous Healing*. "I often heard Dr. Fulford instruct adult patients to crawl as a way of speeding recovery from injuries. "'Go back to this simple movement and you will help the nervous system move beyond any blocks,'" he would say." Your body is constantly renewing itself. All of the skin cells are replaced in five weeks and our skeletal structure is completely regenerated in three months. Body has an amazing ability to regenerate and heal itself!*

In today's world filled with technology and machines, we have forgotten how to naturally use our bodies. Yet we are like trees, we have been provided with everything we need to be healthy. All you need is your body and your loving care! So, why wait till you get to the gym, recognize how wonderful it is that you've been granted an amazing ability to move. The key is not the quantity or location but focused attention, concentration and muscle awareness. Strength will build in your body, if you consciously send the energy to the muscles you are working. BELIEVE that all you need to reach your lifetime potential is already within you!!!

Awaken Your Embryonic Fluidity Movement

♦ <u>Cat and Snake Flow</u>

Purpose: Explore the pleasant and comfortable ways of moving and stretching.

Sequence:

Start on hands and knees. Move your spine in different ways. Arch and round, imagine you are rubbing like an animal against a tree trunk, move your neck and head. Look side-to-side, move like a snake as your hips go to the right, your head moves to the left and vice versa. Now try to make the movement smooth and fluid. Rock your hips side to side, in circles, back and forth and be playful.

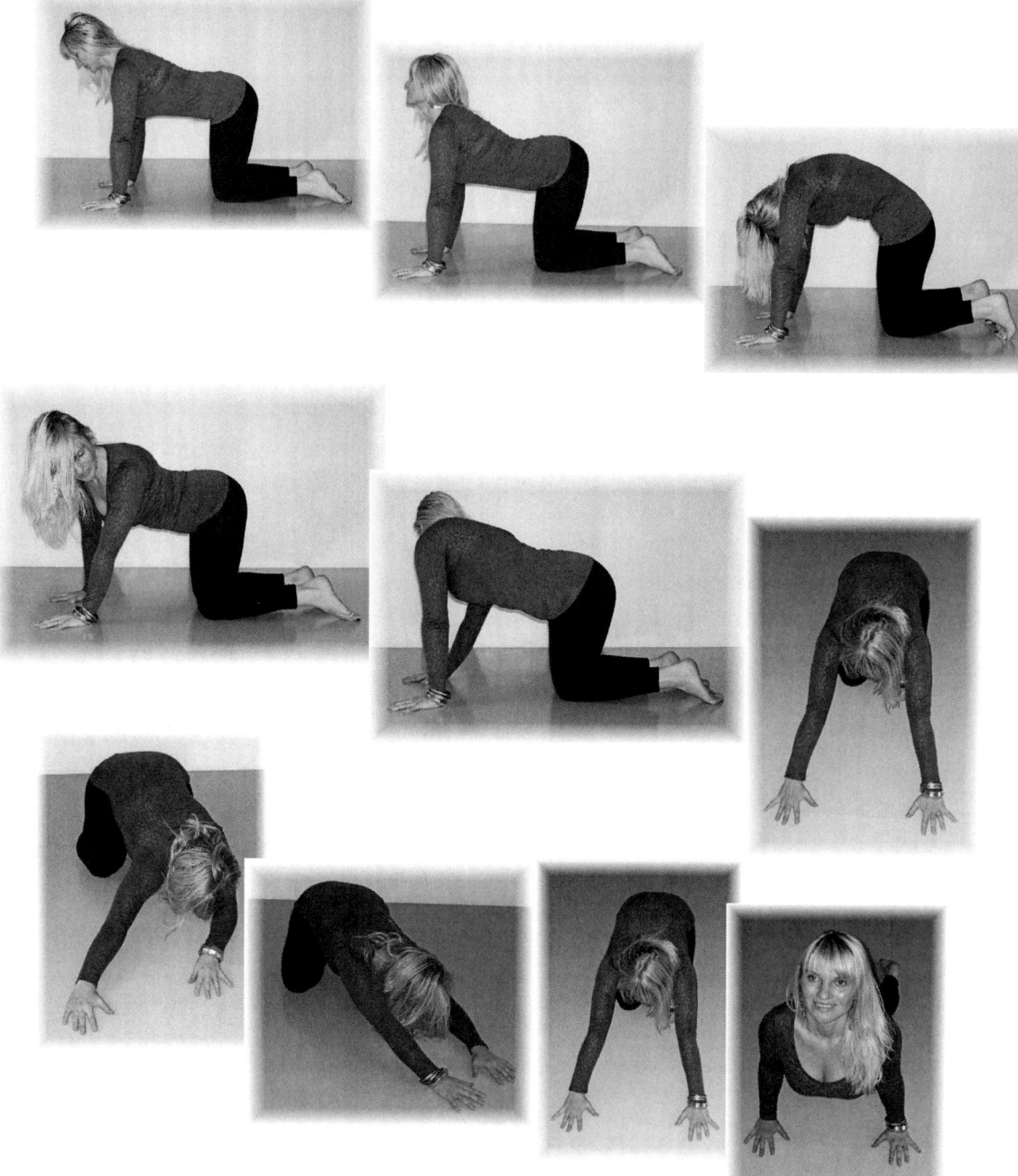

The Heart's Way to Happiness and Health

◆ Floating on Your Back

Purpose: Promotes healing to all joints, develops fluidity and balance.

Sequence:

Lie on your belly. Extend your left arm, bend your right knee and roll on your left side. (You can use your right arm to help you push off the ground.) Simultaneously, lift your legs to the ceiling and roll on your back. Move your arms and legs as if you are swimming in the sky. Be playful; you can roll side to side, open and close your legs, rock your hips side to side, hold your toes like a happy baby and move your legs about. Spend time here for as long as you like. Extend your left arm behind you and roll onto your left side and back onto your belly.

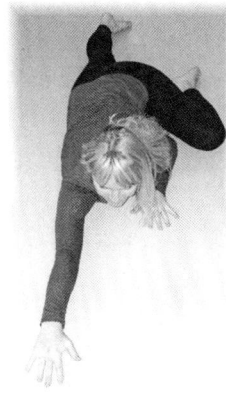
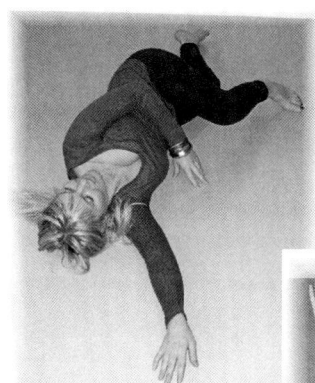
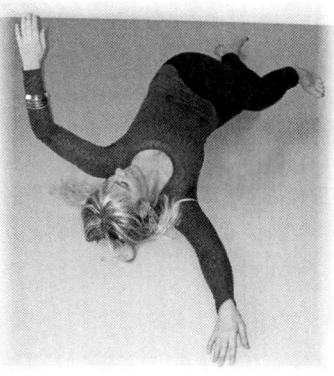
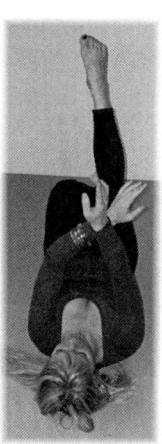

The Heart's Way to Happiness and Health

Extend your right arm, bend your left knee and roll onto your right side and onto your back. Move, flow and play for as long as you like. Repeat rolling from one side to other as many times as you like. Finish by rolling onto your belly.

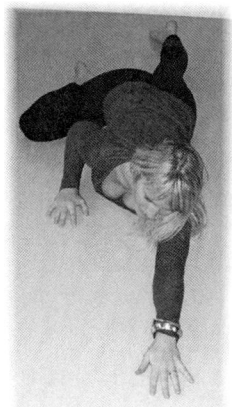

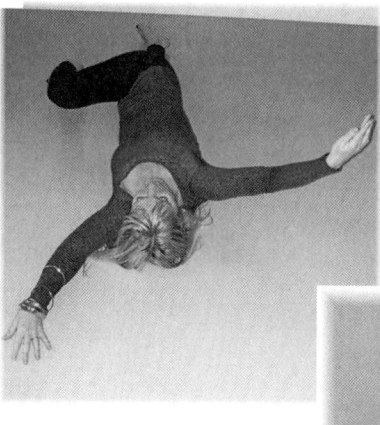

♦ Crawling

Purpose: Improves upper body strength, stimulates healing and releases your hip joints for a fluid and youthful gait.

Sequence:

Lying on the abdomen, bend your right knee and extend your left arm. Bend your left elbow and straighten your right knee as you drag yourself across the floor like an infant. See how slow and how fast can you crawl!

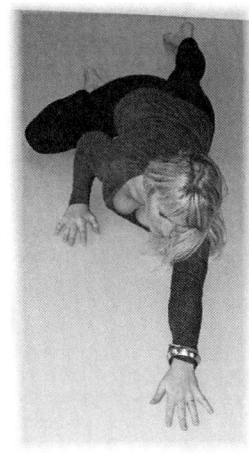
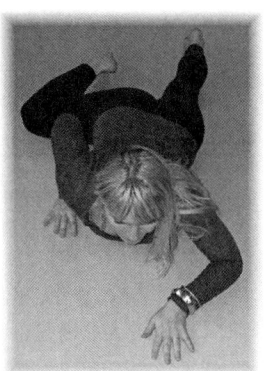
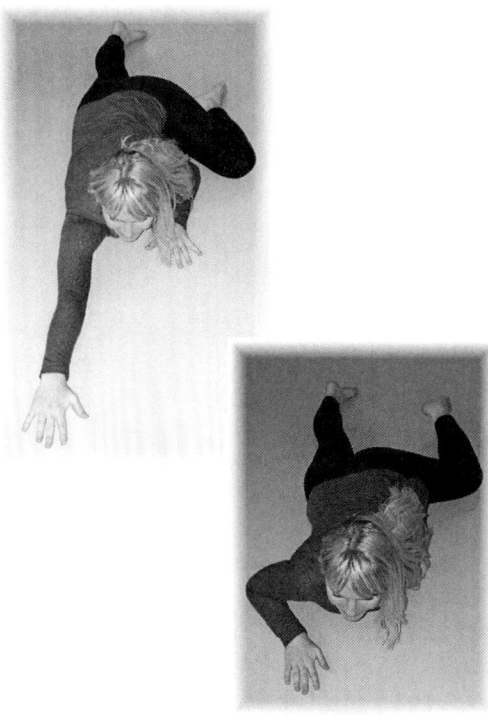

The Heart's Way to Happiness and Health

♦ <u>Walking on Hands and Knees</u>
Purpose: Exploring your joint mobility, agility, balance and strength.

Sequence:
Walk on all fours like a baby across the room.

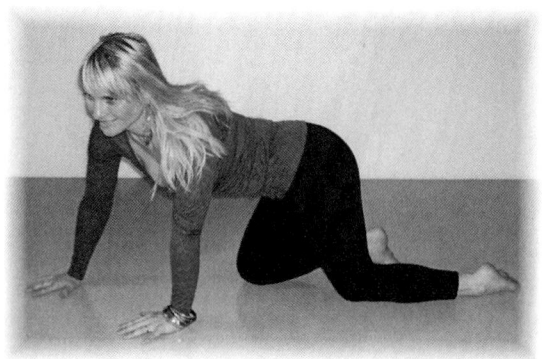

♦ Lower and Rise

Purpose: Getting up from the floor requires the engagement of many muscles. If we do not practice this simple movement daily, our joints will get stiff and we will not know that we are losing our primordial strength to raise and lower ourselves effortlessly from the ground.

Sequence: Practice lowering yourself to the ground and then standing back up. Repeat 4-9 times. Be creative: squat, push up, tippy toe… Use a wall or chair for balance if needed.

Example: Bend one knee and come up to kneeling lunge, then push with your feet and use your legs to stand up, leading with your head. Be creative and seek comfort and strength as you are learning all over again and again how to lower and rise.

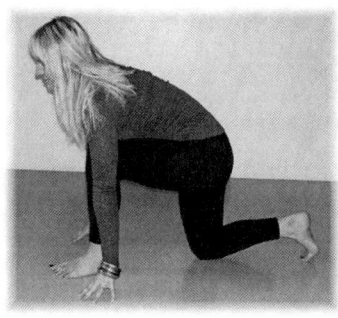
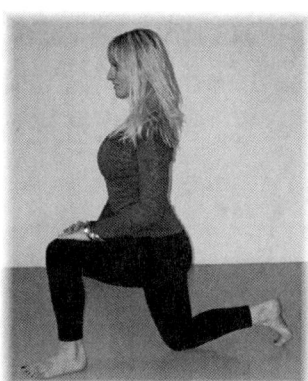
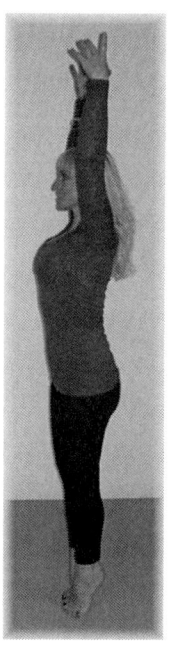

The Heart's Way to Happiness and Health

- <u>Dance, Dance, Dance!</u>

Purpose: Strengthens, tones, streamlines figure, awakens creativity and agility.

- Dance like a child: skip, hop, spin, turn, wiggle, shake your booty! Just move, stop thinking, stop counting, make every move new and fresh, go beyond what you know and what you think is normal for you. Put some music on and have some fun!

- Dance slowly, create your own Tai Chi balancing moves and move with the sounds of the forest or practice by the roar of the ocean.

- Learn belly dancing, a ballroom or another form of dance. It will develop your spatial orientation skills, teach you how to sense and energetically relate to the partner and stimulate your body and brain in new ways.

You should dance! Dance is life, dance is intelligence, dance is your birthright. When you were a child, you would start rocking your hips the instant you heard your favorite music play. Even before you knew how to say your first words, you danced and smiled, because it felt good. What happened, how did we forget? Or we just simply grew up.

Richard Powers, dance historian at the Stanford University states:

"The 21-year study of senior citizens, 75 and older, was led by the Albert Einstein College of Medicine in New York City, funded by the National Institute on Aging, and published in the New England Journal of Medicine. Their method for objectively measuring mental acuity in aging was to monitor rates of dementia, including Alzheimer's disease.

The study wanted to see if any physical or cognitive recreational activities influenced mental acuity. They discovered that some activities had a significant beneficial effect. Other activities had none.

They studied cognitive activities such as reading books, writing for pleasure, doing crossword puzzles, playing cards and playing musical instruments. And they studied physical activities like playing tennis or golf, swimming, bicycling, dancing, walking for exercise and doing housework.

One of the surprises of the study was that almost none of the physical activities appeared to offer any protection against dementia. There can be cardiovascular benefits of course, but the focus of this study was the mind. There was one important exception: the only physical activity to offer protection against dementia was frequent dancing.

Reading - 35% reduced risk of dementia
Bicycling and swimming - 0%

People who played the hardest gained the most: For example, seniors who did crossword puzzles four days a week had a 47% lower risk of dementia than those who did the puzzles once a week.

> *Playing golf - 0%*
> ***Dancing frequently - 76%.***

That was the greatest risk reduction of any activity studied, cognitive or physical."

The excerpt was reprinted with permission.

Feel the Smile in Your Heart – Yoga-and Pilates Program

Why Yoga and Pilates?

- **Keeps your spine and joints youthful.**

Yoga and Pilates is an ideal exercise combination that fuses flexibility with strength. Both disciplines keep your spine flexible and supple, while strengthening the postural muscles that support skeletal alignment.

The photo on the left shows my upper back posture before incorporating yoga and Pilates into my life. With time, yoga, Pilates and mindfulness of my posture throughout the day opened up shoulders and strengthened upper back muscles, which stabilize my scapula. The final result is a broadened back, opened-up shoulders and chest. Also, the stabilized scapula has prevented shoulder injuries.

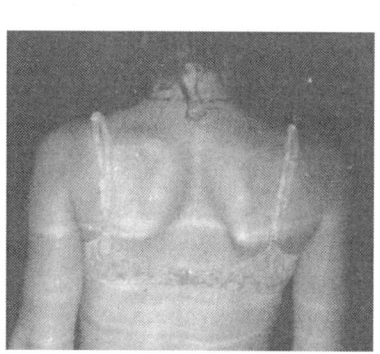
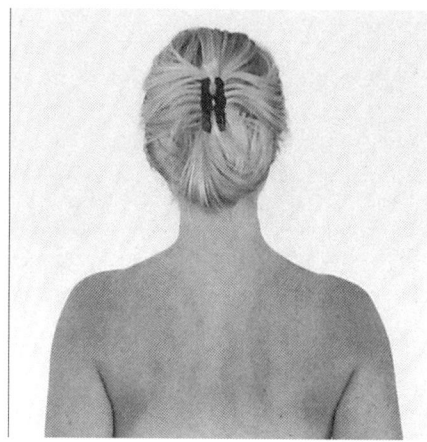

- **Keeps your muscles and connective tissues youthful.**

In the <u>Natural Awakening</u> article "Movement as Medicine" Katy Bowman writes "[a] according to the science journal, *Muscle & Nerve*, it is impossible to determine the age of the muscle by looking at it under the microscope. It can be 18 or 80 year old. What they can tell is the effects of inflexibility and tension that tears and wears the tissue and joints." By keeping our muscles and connective tissue pliable with flexibility exercises and mindful movement, we supply oxygen and nutrients required for cell regeneration, which promotes muscle plasticity, joint health and graceful movement.

If you bend to pick a flower, the muscles in the front of the body, your abdomen and the front of the hips, have to contract, while the muscles in the back of the body, your spinal muscles and back of the hips are lengthening and slowing you down to prevent you from falling. Your muscles have to work in an integrated way as a unit and not as separate body parts to complete even the simplest task.

If the muscles along your spine, in your hips and legs are too tight, then you will have a greater chance of straining your back. You might not be able to bend down to pick up a flower, a child or a grocery bag. If muscles don't have enough tension, that is strength, then they will not be able to bring you to the upright position without hurting your back and you might stumble and fall. Balance between muscle tensile strength and flexibility in opposing muscles groups is very important. Your muscles have to be elastic like bungee cords: stretchy to accomplish the task of bending, yet strong to do it safely and lift you back into the neutral position. Yoga and Pilates train your body in an integrated way by teaching you how to use your body as a whole. It prepares you for daily activities so that you can enjoy them to your fullest by combining dynamic poses with flexibility to maintain and return to the balanced neutral alignment. The beauty of yoga and Pilates is that no matter what your age is, you will be able to do at least some yoga poses and Pilates exercises. And the earlier you start, the easier it will be for you to keep it up.

- **Keeps your voice and skin youthful.**

Breathing exercises strengthen and expand your lungs, improve skin tone and eliminate toxic waste. Every action from digestion to muscle contraction requires oxygen. Yoga and Pilates teach you how to breathe deeply and retrain yourself from shallow upper chest breathing.

- **Keeps your mind youthful.**

Yoga and Pilates requires focused attention and awareness, which improves your physical balance and concentration of the mind. Breathing exercises rejuvenates brain cells, promotes restful sleep and positive attitude.

- **Keeps you youthful inside out.**

Yoga is a 5,000 year old healing art that harmonizes emotions, awakens our creativity, intuition and develops spiritual realization of our unity to everything in the universe.

Tip 1: Practice yoga and Pilates at least 3 times a week. If you are a beginner, start with 20-minutes and build-up to 1-hour practice.

Tip 2: Invest into buying yourself a yoga mat. Because you practice with bare feet, mat will keep your feet from sliding and you will feel more grounded.

Tip 3: Move with awareness and feeling. Slow and controlled movements will give you more positive results. Pay complete attention to what you are doing. Be focused and in tune with your body. Turn off your cell phone and set aside time to focus attention on your body, mind and breath. You will feel that you are ready for the world with renewed enthusiasm and energy, if you take the time to do this.

Caution: Discontinue any exercise if you experience pain or discomfort.

Neck Release

If you notice that you have a tight neck, it is beneficial to do gentle neck stretches before you begin yoga and Pilates or perform neck stretches sometime during your day to help release tension. Perform the following neck stretches seated in a chair. Place your feet flat on the floor. Relax your shoulders and neck while keeping your head aligned and centered over your body.

Caution: Consult your physician before doing neck stretches and exercises, if you have any neck problems or pain.

- <u>Neck Circles</u>

Relax your neck and shoulders. Make sure your head is directly aligned and centered over your body. Bring your right ear to your right shoulder, then gently roll your head down toward your chest and over the other shoulder. Continue by gently rolling your head backward to complete the circle. Roll a few times in one direction, then return your head to neutral and repeat in the opposite direction.

Awareness: Perform this experiment: sit in a chair, place your awareness in your face and turn your head to the left to look over your left shoulder, then over the right shoulder. Repeat this several times. Now perform the same head movements, however, this time bring your awareness to the back of your head. Which way feels more free to you? We often keep our head in a head forward position, by brining more awareness to the back of the head as we move during the day, helps us with head-neck-spine alignment.

♦ <u>Neck Extensors (back of the neck)</u>

Place one hand on the back of your head and one hand under your chin. Roll your head down towards your chest. You can gently assist at the end of each stretch by pressing lightly down with your top hand on your head. Hold for 2 seconds. Return to neutral position. Repeat 5 times. Now switch hands and repeat 5 times with the other hand on top.

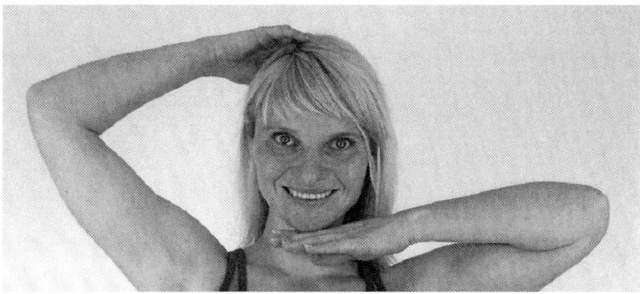

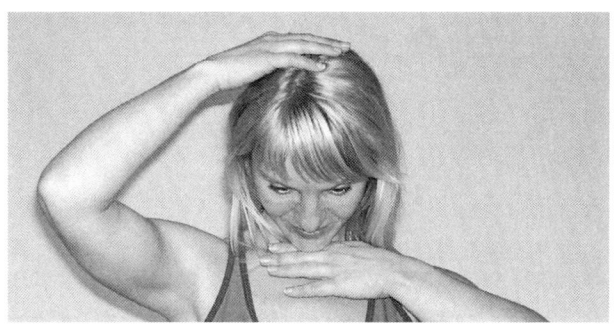

The Heart's Way to Happiness and Health

- ♦ <u>Neck Flexors (front of the neck)</u>

Place your fingers along your jawbone. Then roll your head straight back, chin straight up. You can gently assist the stretch by pressing with your fingers. Hold for 2 seconds, return to neutral position and repeat 5 times. This exercise also tones muscles in front of the neck.

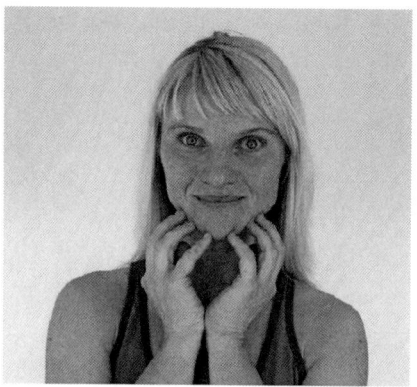

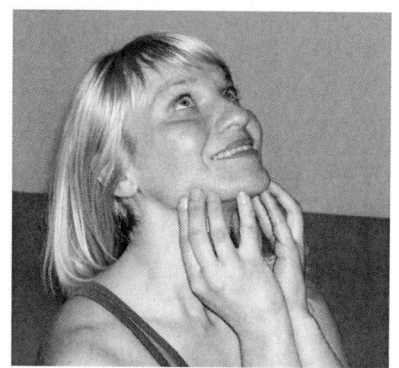

- Neck Lateral Flexors (side of the neck)

Place right hand on the left side of your head. Tilt your head to the right toward your right shoulder. Point your nose slightly downward. Feel the stretch on the left side of the neck. Hold for 15 seconds. Slowly come back to center and repeat one more time. Now do the other side.

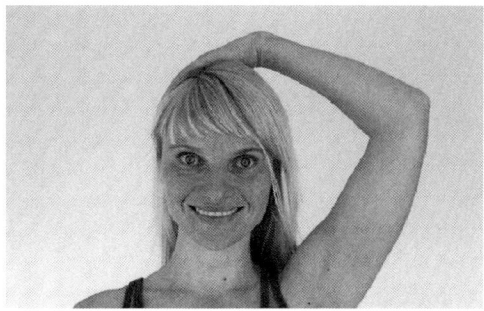

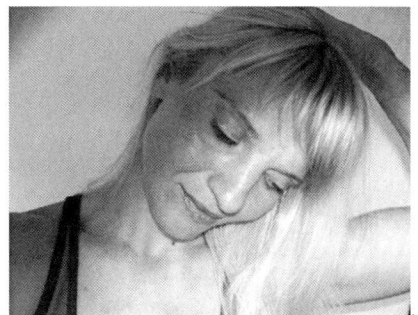

The Heart's Way to Happiness and Health

- Neck Flexor Oblique Stretch

Place your right hand's index and middle fingers on the left side of the back of the head. Turn your face 45 degrees to the right and bring your head down at a 45 degree angle. Gently assist the stretch by pressing with your fingers on the back of the head. You will feel the stretch on the left side of the back of the neck in the muscle that attaches your scapula to the cervical spine. Hold for 15 seconds and slowly lift your head and come back to neutral. Now repeat on the other side.

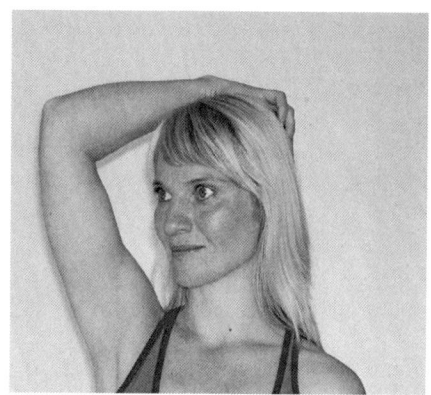

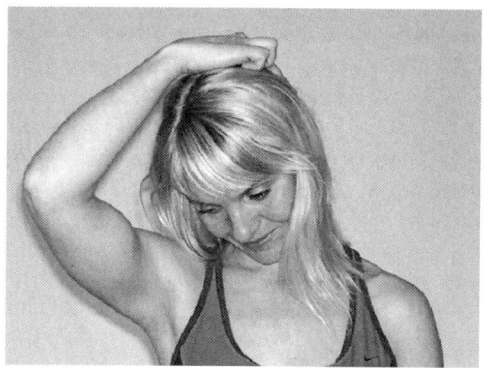

♦ Meditation

Purpose: Centering and relaxing mind and body.

Sequence:

1. Sit crossed-legged. Widen your buttocks by creating more space between your sitting bones, the bones in your buttocks. Place your right hand under your right buttock and roll the buttock out to the side, then do the same on the left side. Evenly distribute your weight on both sitting bones. Feel yourself connecting through your roots, your sit bones, into the ground, spinal column bones like blocks stacked vertically over each other. Lift chest to free your abdomen for breathing, keep shoulders broad, yet relaxed, with the crown of your head freely floating upwards. Rest your hands in the lap, with palms up and thumbs gently connecting to your index fingers. Relax your hands.

2. Close your eyes, relax your jaw, scalp and shoulders. Set all everything aside, let your complete attention be on your breathing. Breathe in through your nose and breathe out through your nose, breathe in, breathe out… Feel your breathing, listen to your breathing. If your mind wonders away, gently direct it back to breathing, go deeper and deeper into relaxation with each breath. Meditate for as long as you like, try to access silence within, be so still and peaceful that a bird might want to land on you.

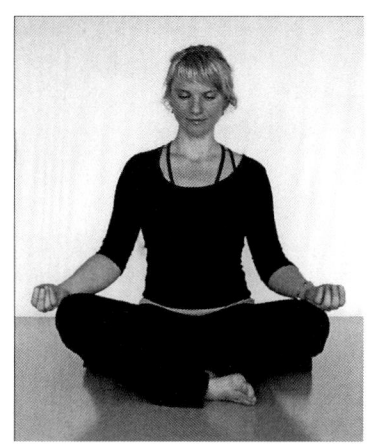

3. Bring palms together and set a goal for your practice. It can be physical, such as: I want to improve flexibility in my hips; or it can be more mental, such as: I want practice the joy in my heart throughout my workout. Say your focus mentally to yourself and also visualize yourself doing what you intend. Feel as if you have already reached your focus.

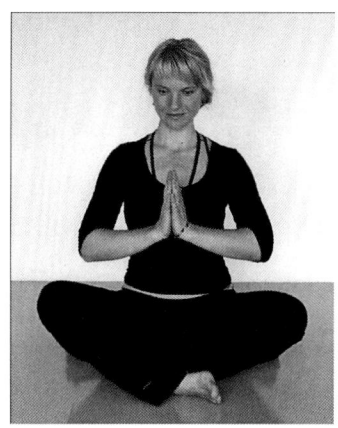

Awareness: *Are you able to relax your hips and float your spine effortlessly upwards? How about, if you sit on the blanket or a thick book? Does this help your back and hips? If you still not comfortable, begin seated in a chair.*

The Heart's Way to Happiness and Health

♦ Shoulder and Upper Back Release

Bring your arms at the sides. Inhale and shrug your shoulders up to your ears, exhale and release your shoulders down by gliding your scapula down the back. Repeat 5 times.

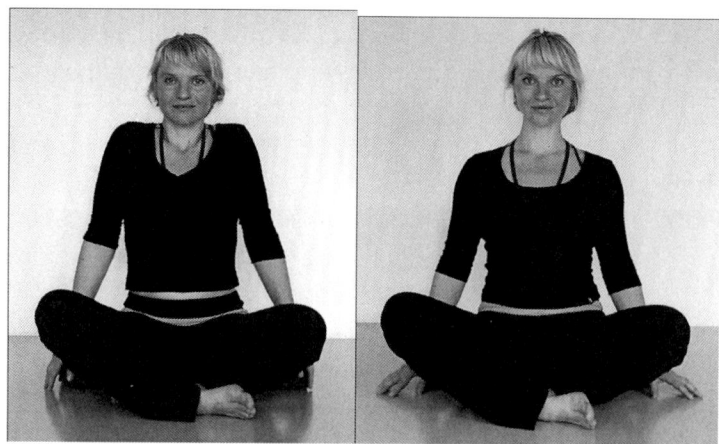

♦ Seated Spine Lengthener

Purpose: Activates breathing muscles, expands chest, lengthens and decompresses the spine.

Sequence:

1. Inhale, turn your palms out, glide the scapula down your back as if you are trying to put your shoulder blades into your back pockets, look upwards and lift your arms up from your sides. Stretch and lengthen through the sides of your body, at the same time feel the rooting into the ground through the sit bones.

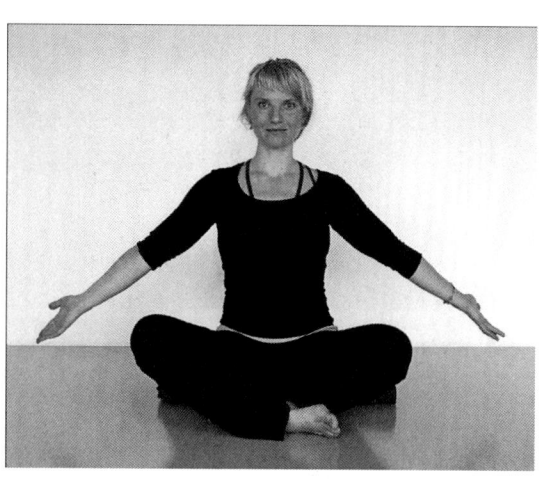
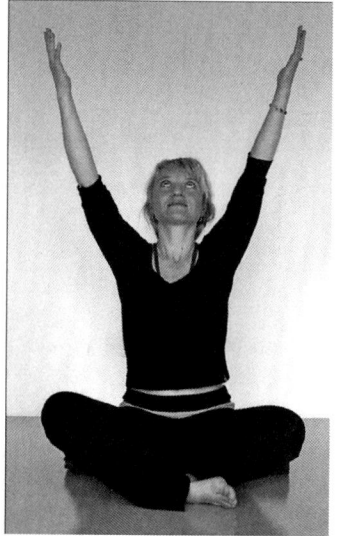

The Heart's Way to Happiness and Health

2. Exhale, lower your arms back down at your sides and nod your chin down. Repeat the breathing, lifting and lowering your arms 5 times.

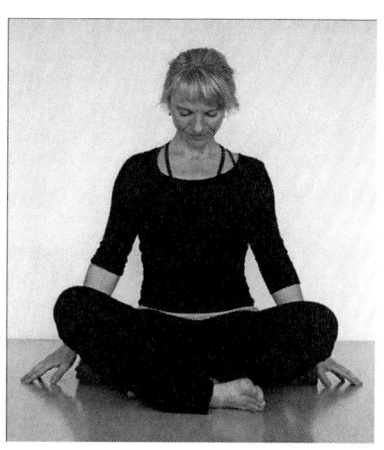

Awareness: *Be mindful which leg is crossed in front. If you always prefer your one side, then make sure to switch legs and practice with the other leg in front.*

3. On the fifth time clasp your hands over your head. Inhale and lengthen your spine; exhale, side bend to the right, look upward toward your left upper arm bone. Inhale, come back up, exhale and side bend to the left, look upward to your right upper arm bone.

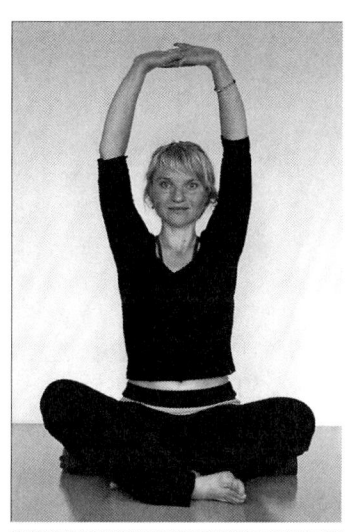
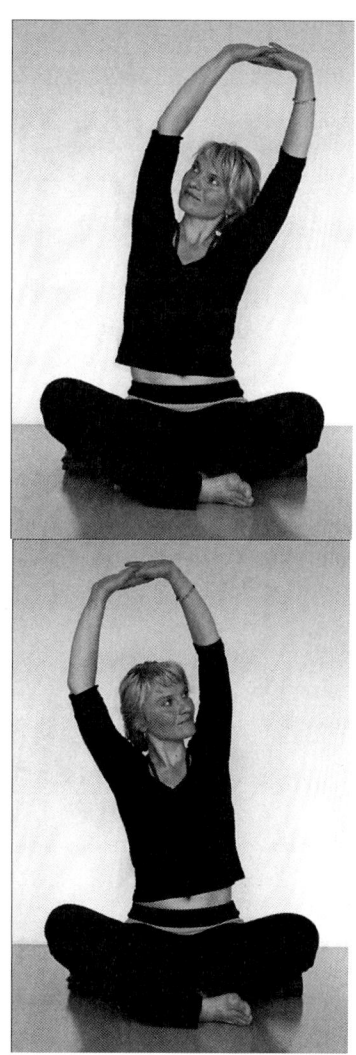
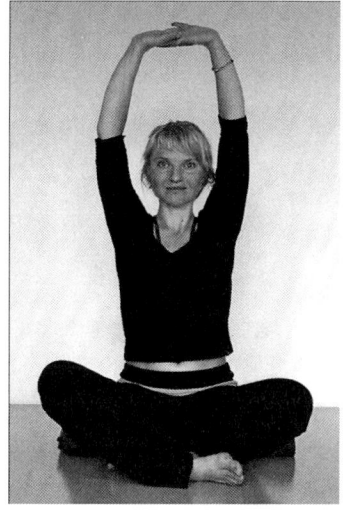

The Heart's Way to Happiness and Health

4. Inhale, come back up to the center. Exhale and twist to your right, inhale, come back to the center, exhale and twist to your left, inhale, come back to the center.

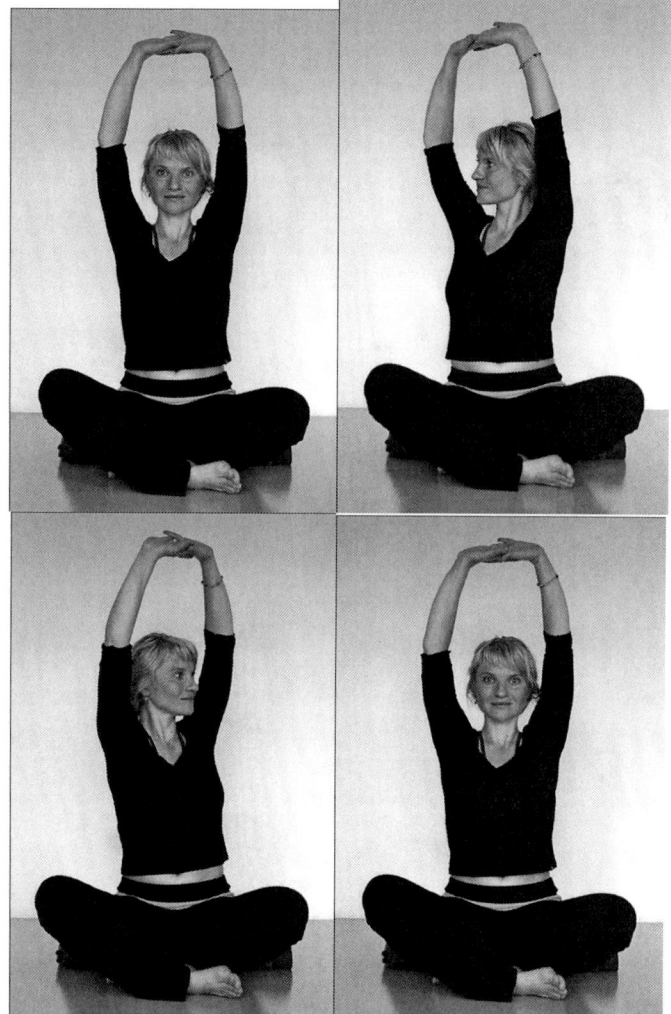

Awareness: *Experiment with arm positioning and explore the comfort of your shoulders and wrists. Try the same sequence with hands unclasped and elbows bent.*

5. Inhale, separate your hands, exhale and weightlessly float your arm down to rest at your sides. Circle your shoulders one way a few times then the other way. Finish by circling once to the back to keep your shoulders open.

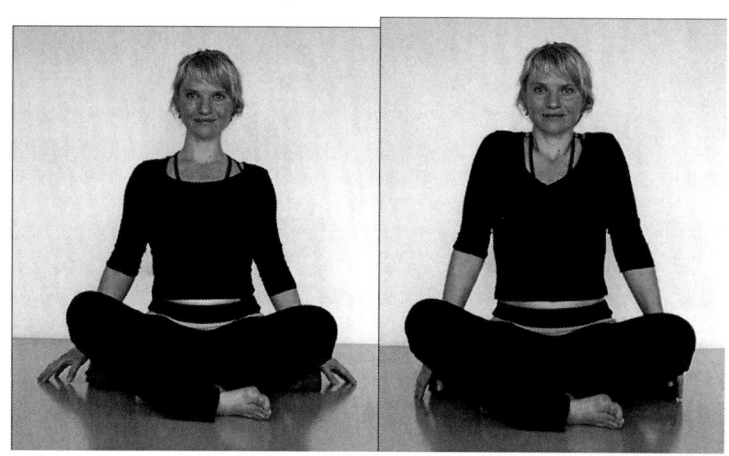

6. Bring palms together and feel after effects of the spine lengthener. Melt your shoulders, relax groin and hips, lower your gaze or close your eyes and breathe into your belly.

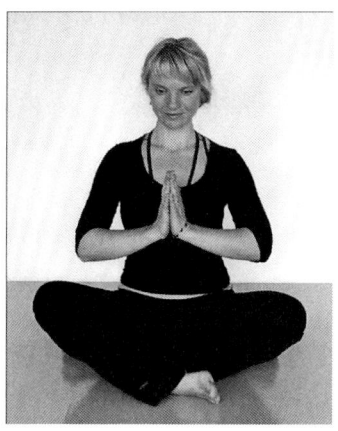

Visual: *Drape your thighs down as if they are light as silk.*

The Heart's Way to Happiness and Health

♦ Cat and Cow:

Purpose: Improves spine flexibility, tones abdominals, prevents back pain and stretches feet.

Sequence:
1. Start on all fours, bringing hands under the shoulders and the knees under the hips. Open your fingers apart. Keep your spine neutral, lower back slightly arched. Imagine an arrow shooting straight from the crown of your head and directly back from the tailbone.

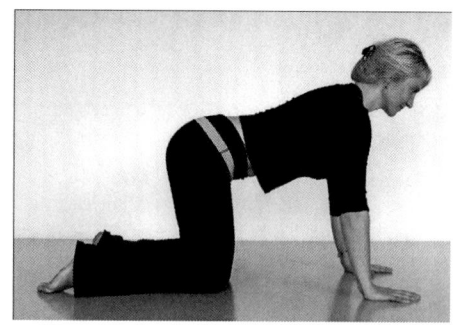

2. Inhale and arch your lower back gently, draw your ribcage forward and up. Lift your chest and gaze upwards to Cow pose.

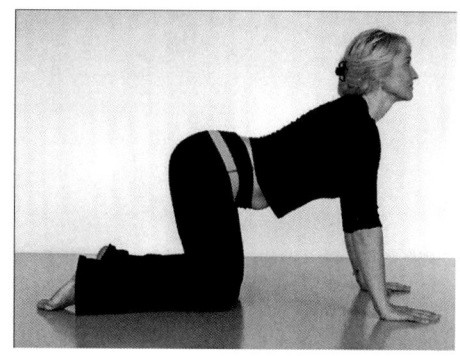

3. Exhale, round your back to Cat stretch. Tighten your abdominals, release your head down, broaden upper back and feel the stretch between your shoulder blades.

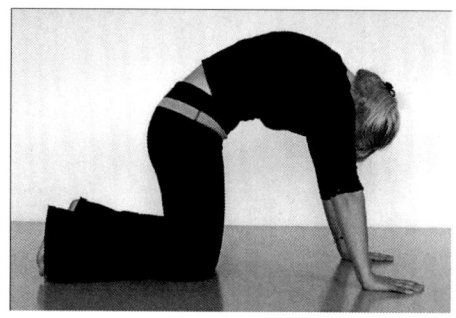

4. Repeat arching and rounding 5-10 times.

Awareness: *Begin the movement from your tailbone, move vertebra by vertebra, last part to lift or lower is you head.*

◆ <u>Child's Pose</u>

Purpose: Gently stretch hips, back and ankles.

Sequence:
1. Start kneeling on the ground. Place hands in front of the shoulders. Bring the big toes together and separate your heels slightly apart. Knees about hip distance apart. Inhale.

2. Exhale and bring your hips to the heels. Straighten your arms in front of your body and lengthen your torso. If it is comfortable, relax your head by placing your hairline on the floor. Keep the back of your neck long. Pause and breathe into your lower back and hips for 5 deep breaths.

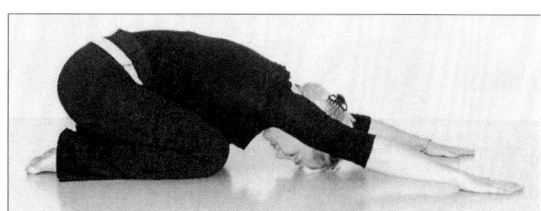

Modifications:
For the comfort of your shoulders, bend and rest your elbows on the ground with elbows wider than your shoulders.

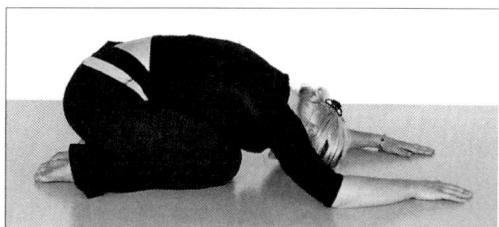

Or place your hands at the sides of your feet with your palms up to the sky and breathe.

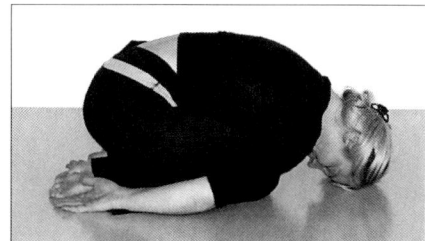

♦ Downward Facing Dog

Purpose: Strengthens core, legs and arms. Stretches shoulders, the back of the upper and lower legs.

Sequence:

1. Kneel on the ground with your knees under your hips and hands a little in front of the shoulders. Spread your fingers.

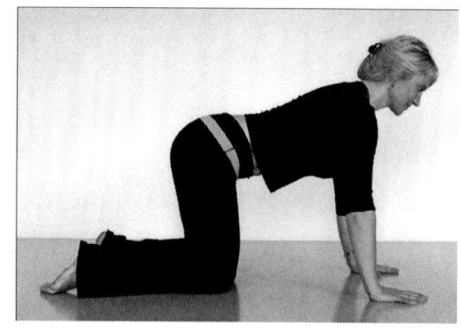

Hand Detail:
Connect through every pad of your finger.

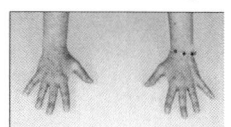

2. Curl the toes under, exhale and lift your knees off the ground, reaching your hips back and up, into Downward Facing Dog.

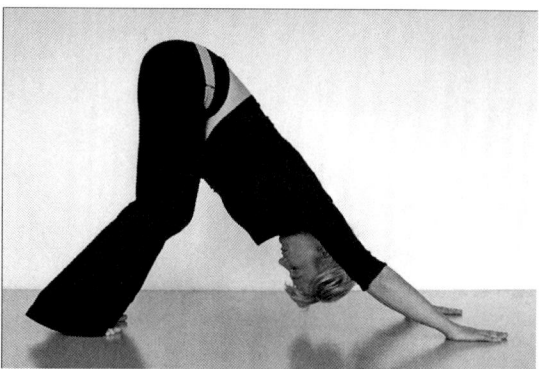

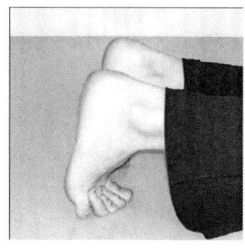

Detail:
Curl toes under. Prevent your ankles from rolling out by keeping inner edges of your feet parallel.

Special Notes: Bend knees slightly, heels off the ground, push the floor away from you with your hands and lift sit bones up to the ceiling and then back towards the back wall. Keep full connection through your hands and feel even weight between your hands and feet. Widen shoulder blades broad across your back and glide them upwards toward your hips. Feel the lengthening in the triceps of your upper arms and up through your spine to create weightlessness in the shoulders. Relax the neck by keeping your ears in line with your upper arm bones.

3. Press your heels to the ground and straighten your knees

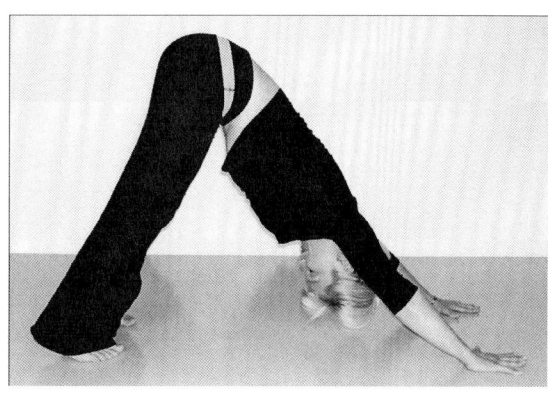

Special Notes: *Now, as you are straightening the knees, maintain lengthened spine, activate your upper thighs and press them to the back wall. Gradually you will be able to lower your heels down to the ground and straighten knees. However, you should sustain the lengthened spine throughout the pose. If it is too difficult, try lowering your right heel to the ground first, as your left knee is bent, then your left heel to the ground and the right knee is bent. Alternate them until you get more limber to lower both heels to the ground.*

4. Lower your knees and bring your hips back to Child's pose, p. 48.

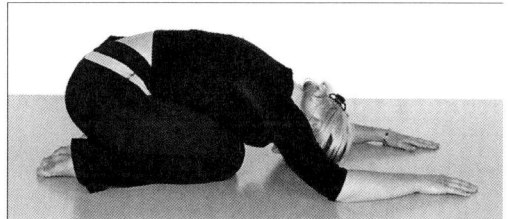

Puppy - Downward Facing Dog Modification:
Knees bent on the ground, elbows on the floor, shoulders wide. Feel how your hips are reaching back behind you. Lower back is slightly arched in neutral curves. Be careful not to let your ribcage drop toward the floor and put pressure in your lower or middle back. To prevent that, draw your ribs slightly up and in.

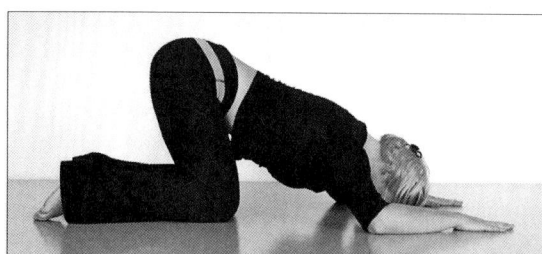

To achieve more spine lengthening action, curl toes under and straighten arms to the front as you push the floor away from you with your hands. Activate abdominals and reach your hips back.

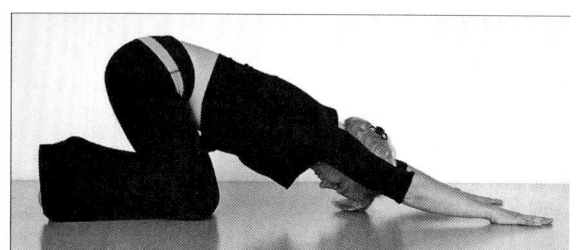

♦ <u>Downward Facing Dog to Upward Facing Dog</u>

Purpose: Strengthens core, legs and arms. Upward Facing Dog stretches shoulders, chest and abdomen. Downward Facing Dog stretches shoulders, the back of the upper and lower legs.

Sequence:
1. Begin on your hands and knees. Exhale and lift your hips back to Downward Facing Dog, inhale and bring hips forward, expand chest to Upward Facing Dog, exhale and lift your hips back to Downward Facing Dog. Repeat flowing from Downward Facing Dog to Upward Facing Dog 3-4 times.

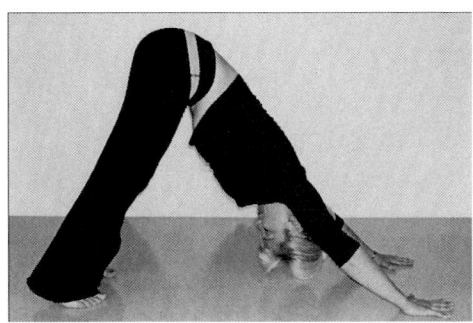 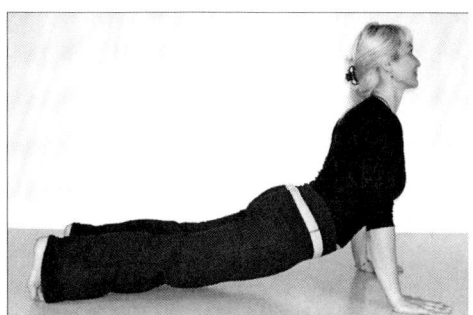

Special Notes for Upward Facing Dog: *Rotate your legs slightly inward at the hip joints. This action opens the sacrum. Tuck your pubic bone slightly in to lengthen and protect your lower back. Lift your breast bone, broaden upper back and relax shoulders down. Arms straight but make sure not to lock your elbows. Keep your back of the neck long. To ease your back and wrists, instead of Upward Facing Dog perform Cobra pose p. 88.*

♦ Kneeling Lunge

Purpose: Stretches front of the hips and inner thigh/groin area. Strengthens legs, core and arms.

Sequence:

1. From Downward Facing Dog, lower knees to the ground, step your right foot between your hands. Align your right knee with your toes and point your knee and toes straight ahead. Reach your left leg as far back as is comfortable for your knees. Keeping your left foot in line with the knee, rotate the top of the left foot and shin directly to the ground.

Tip: You can start kneeling on the folded blanket to cushion your knees.

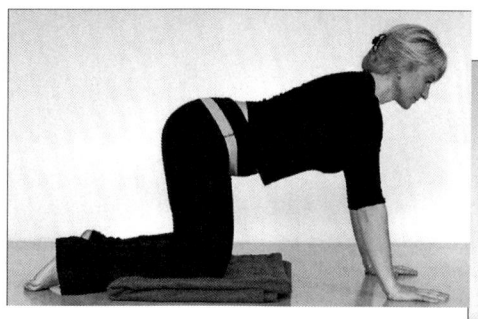
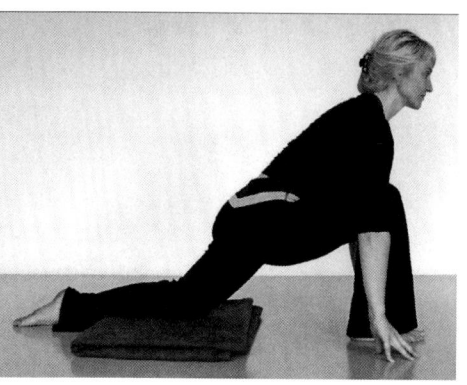

2. Take your hands on the hips and level your hips. Draw your left hip forward and right hip back to level your hips. Tuck pubic bone slightly in to lengthen lower back and prevent lower back from overarching. Shift your hips forward. Expand chest and open shoulders. Hold for 3-5 breaths.

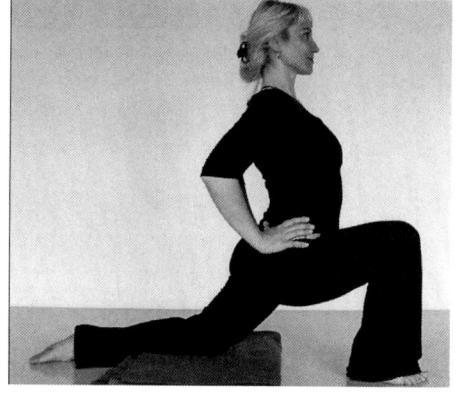

3. Exhale and lower your arms down to the ground, step right foot back to change legs.

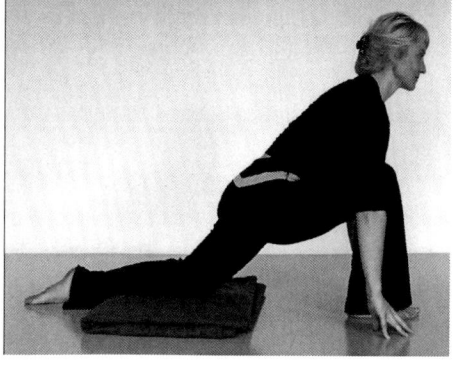
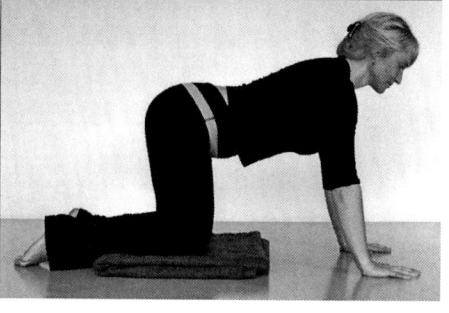

The Heart's Way to Happiness and Health

Modification:
To avoid pulling the back knee, keep the back knee more at a 90-degree angle. You can also place blocks under your hands.

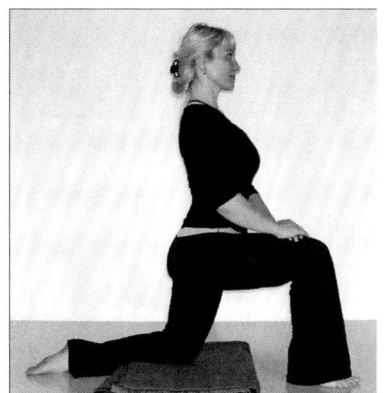 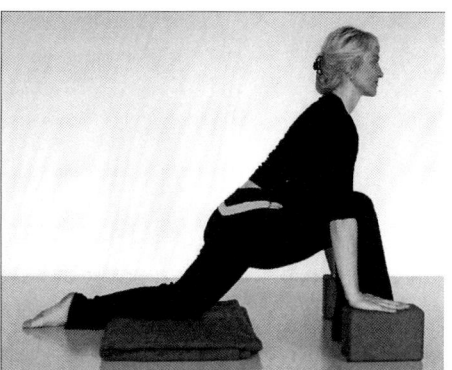

<u>**Caution:**</u> Don't ignore knee pain; discontinue any pose if it doesn't feel right.

Advanced modification:
Inhale and lift your arms up, palms facing each other, and palms together or apart.

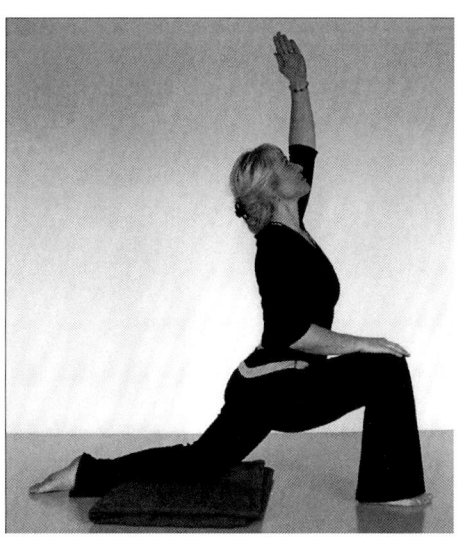 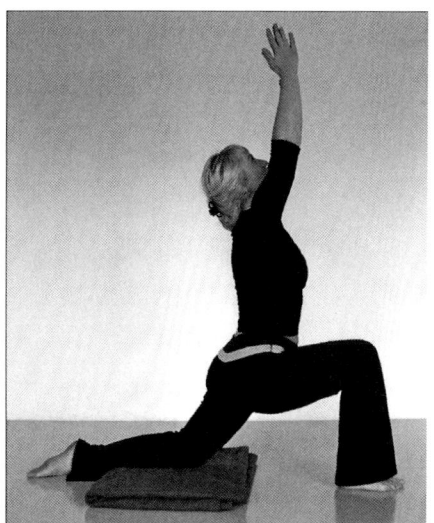

Special Notes: *Keep pelvis gently tucking in to keep lower back lengthened and protected.*

The Heart's Way to Happiness and Health

- <u>Push-ups</u>

Purpose: Strengthens core, chest and arms.

Sequence:

1. Start in the push-up position. Hands under the shoulders, knees off the ground, feet hip distance apart, legs straight. Keep your abdominals active.

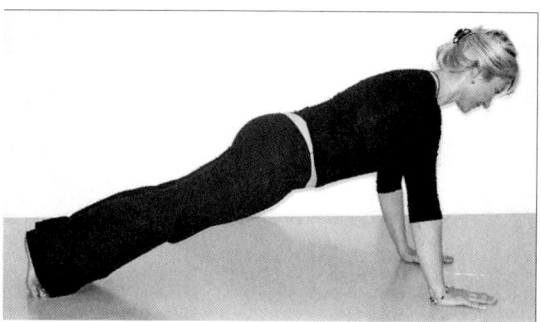

2. Inhale and bend your elbows down, point your elbows straight back and keep them close to your body. Lower your chest straight down, between your hands, hover above the ground. Aim your chest and not your chin between your hands.

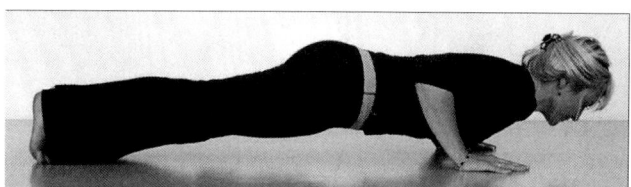

3. Without resting in the hover position, exhale and push straight up as you straighten your arms. Perform 12-20 push-ups.

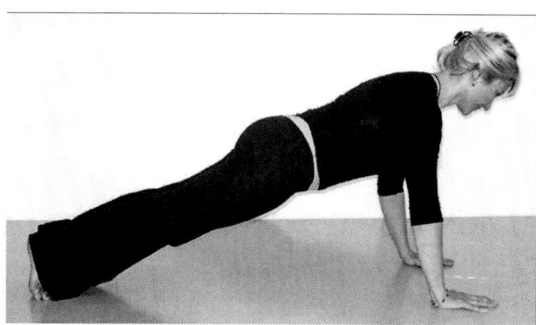

Beginner's modification:
1. Do push-ups on your knees.

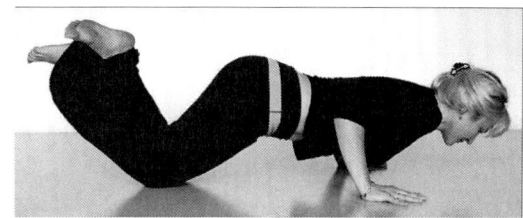

2. Or keep your hips up. You can place a blanket under your knees to cushion them.

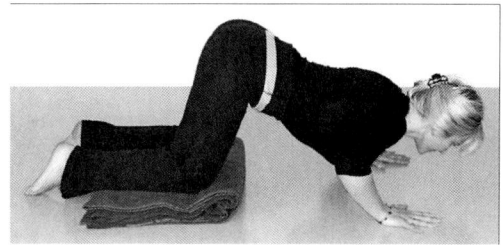

3. If these are still too difficult, try to perform push-ups against the wall.

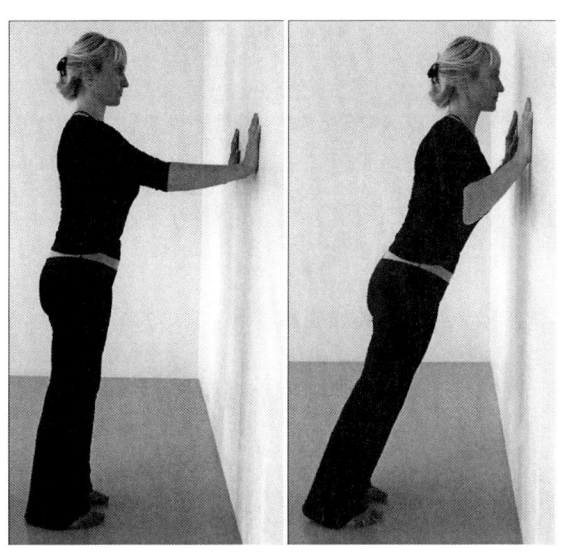

***Special Notes:** The hands under the shoulders or closer than your shoulders works your triceps. Widen your hands and your chest will work more.*

Caution: Skip push-ups, if it bothers your back, shoulders or wrists.

4. After doing push-ups, walk your hands back into Forward Bend pose. Inhale, lengthen your spine, exhale and bend deeper at the creases in the front of your hips as you are straightening your knees, activating your frontal thighs and lifting sit bones up to the ceiling. Try to keep your hips over the front part of your heels. Your knees can bend slightly as you touch the ground with your hands or hold your elbows in the opposite hand to release upper back. Relax your neck. Breathe.

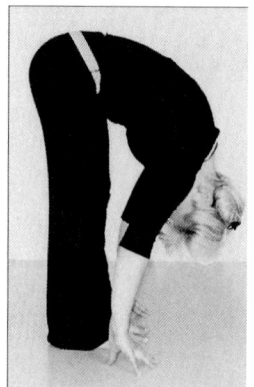 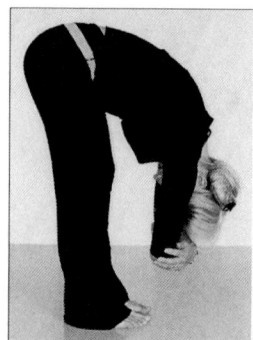

5. Release elbows, engage your abdominals and on your next inhale, slowly roll spine vertebra by vertebra to standing into Mountain pose; the last part to come up is the head.

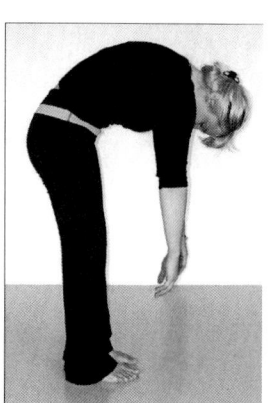 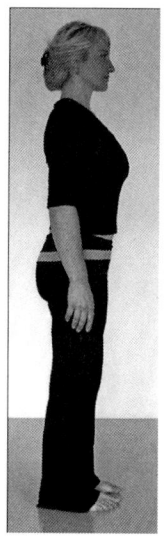

♦ <u>Mountain Pose</u>

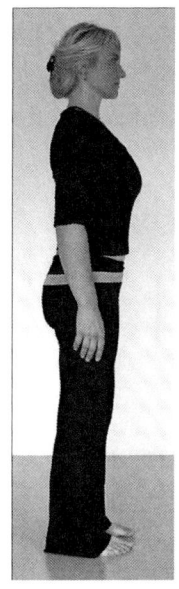

Awareness: *Sometimes it takes a lot of effort to stand in the proper posture, because you are not used to it and what is correct might first seem awkward. See which points of standing tall like a mountain makes sense to your body:*

- *Feet hip distance apart and parallel or big toes together and heels slightly apart.*

- *Knees facing in the same direction as your toes.*

- *Even connection through the whole foot to the ground. Feel balanced between the inner and outer arches of your feet.*

- *Rotate your upper leg bones inward a little, so that you feel you are creating more space in your sacrum.*

- *Unlock your knees.*

- *Tone your lower abdominals.*

- *Lift chest yet don't let your ribs protrude or stick out.*

- *Widen from the tips of your shoulders; keep clavicles parallel to the ground. Relax muscles under your armpits; feel your arms are just hanging loosely like a coat on the coat hanger.*

- *Lengthen the back of the neck. Feel the connection to the sky with the crown of your head.*

♦ Shoulder Rotations

Purpose: Stimulates smooth shoulder function and stretches chest.

Sequence:
1. Hold a strap or belt in front of your body. Pull the strap apart with your hands, lift strap over you head, lower strap behind you feeling a stretch in your shoulders and chest.
2. Lift the strap back up and lower strap in front of the body.
3. Repeat 5-8 times.

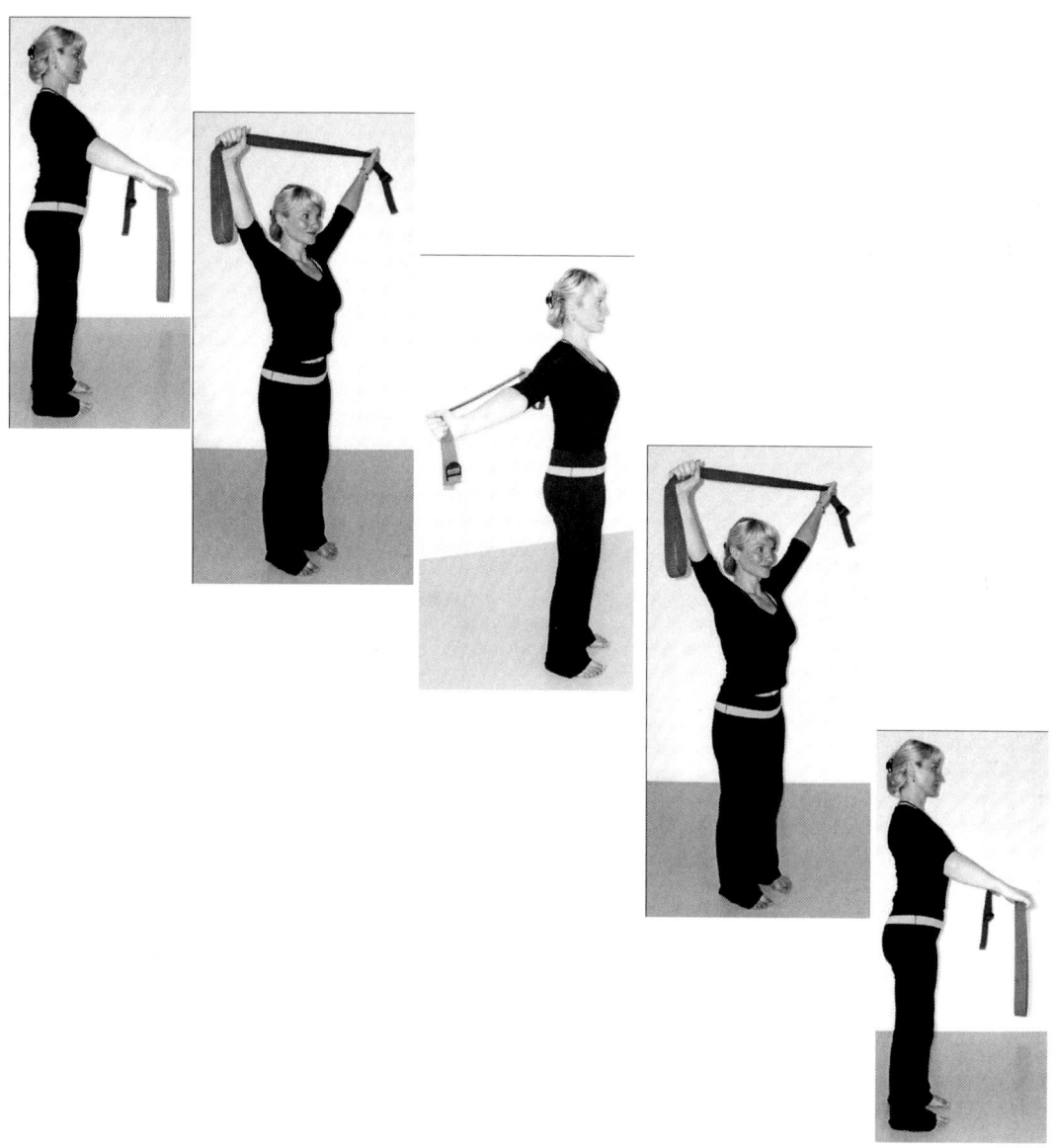

- ### Balance to Chair Pose

Purpose: Strengthens legs, ankles, feet, core and arms. Improves balance.

Sequence:

1. Stand in Prayer position. Inhale and sweep your arms to the sides and upward. Lead with the crown of your head to lift your heels and balance on the balls of your feet. Feet parallel to keep heels from rolling out.
2. Exhale, slowly lower your heels down and squat into Chair pose. Bend your knees and reach your hips back, turn your upper thighs slightly inward to broaden your sacrum. Lower back lengthened and supported with your abdominal muscles, chest open, knees parallel and facing forward in line with your feet. Gaze slightly upward towards your hands with the back of your neck long.
3. Press into your feet, engage abdominals, inhale and straighten yourself up. Activate your legs, tuck pubic bone slightly in, look upwards and comfortably arch backwards. Your hands can be together or they can be shoulder width apart and a little to the front of shoulders.
4. Exhale, come to standing tall, palms together at the heart center with thumbs resting near sternum, shoulders broad and chest expanded. Slightly look downward. Pause feeling the sensations and energy this sequence stimulates through your body.
5. Repeat from beginning 3-4 times.

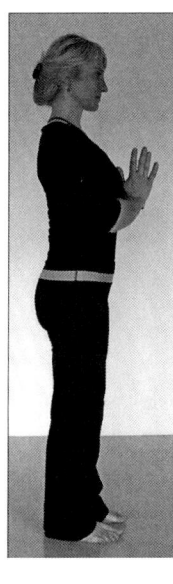
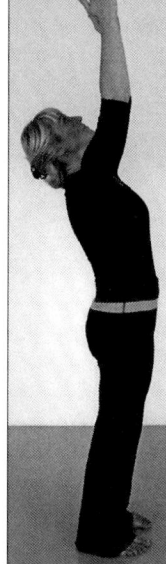
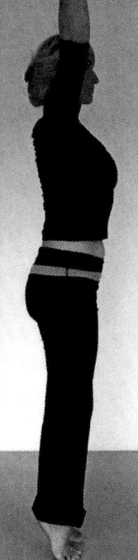
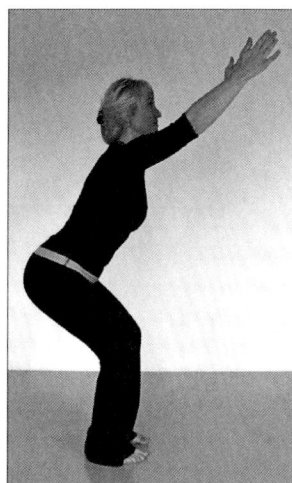
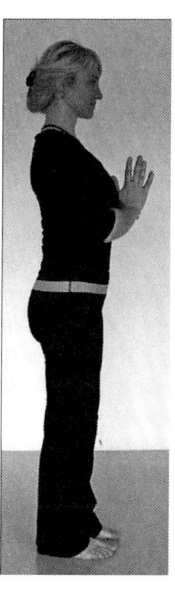

The Heart's Way to Happiness and Health

♦ Warrior I to Proud Warrior to Triangle to Side Angle Bend

Purpose: All poses open chest and shoulders, aligns the spine and strengthen feet, legs, core and arms. Warrior I stretches calves, front of the hips and chest. Proud Warrior/Warrior II stretches groin and legs. Triangle pose stretches calves, back of the legs, hips and groin. Side Angle Bend stretches groin and side of the waist.

Sequence:
1. Stand in a Five Pointed Star. Outstretch your arms to the sides and step your feet about 3 to 5 feet apart so that your feet are approximately under your wrists. Feel the line running from the crown of your head to your pelvic floor. You might need to gently tuck your pubic bone forward to create a lengthened, neutral lower back. Activate abdominals to support your spine.

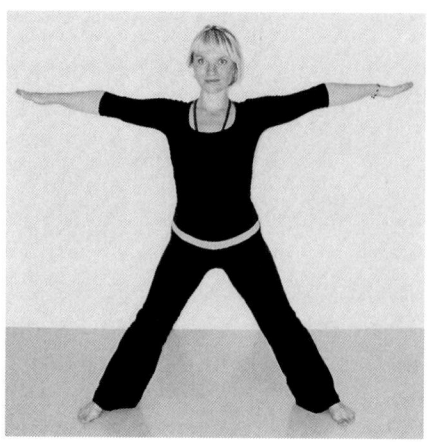

Awareness: Experiment with how far apart you open your legs. Your stance will greatly influence how you experience each pose.

2. Rotate your left foot slightly to the right (inward) and your right foot 90 degrees to the right. Your heels should be aligned throughout the following sequence.

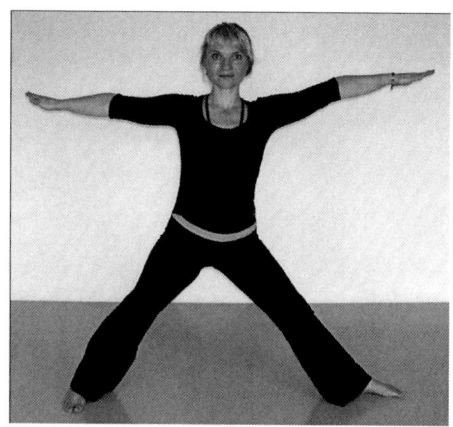

3. Place your hands on your hips and rotate torso and hips as much as is comfortable to the right, bend your right knee.

4. Inhale and lift arms upwards into Warrior I pose. Ground your left heel to the floor and lift up through your left thigh, torso, through your arms and up into your small fingers. Press your right front heel into the ground to lift your torso up and away from the frontal thigh. Feel the shoulder blades broad across your back and gliding down toward your tailbone. Look upwards. Hold for 2-3 breaths.

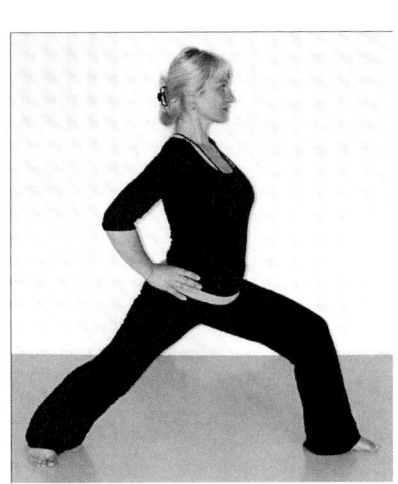 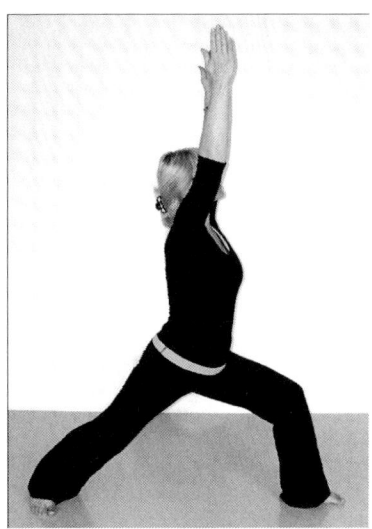

5. Flow into Proud Warrior or Warrior II. Open your pelvis to the left. Simultaneously, inhale and open your arms out to your sides parallel to the ground, expand your chest, keep shoulder blades broad across your back, shoulders down, arms actively engaged and your palms rotated down at your forearms and not at your shoulders. Work your legs by keeping your right thigh rotating outward, so that your right knee is pointing in the same direction as your foot and in line with your second toe. Activate your left leg by grounding into the outer edge of the left foot. Keep your head up in line with pelvic floor. Gaze ahead beyond your right index finger. Breathe for 2-3 breaths.

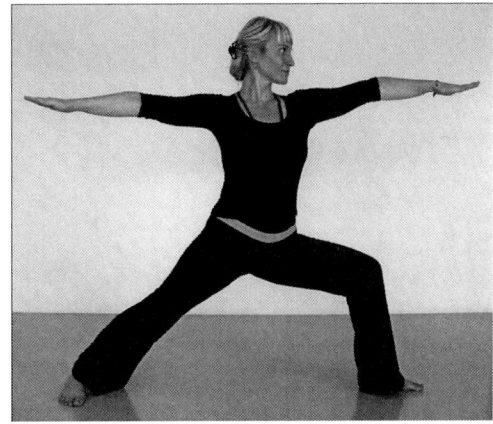

6. Flow into Triangle pose. Press into your feet and straighten your right knee. Activate your legs by keeping your frontal thigh muscles engaged and lifting your kneecaps up your legs yet keep knees unlocked. Inhale, shift your hips to the left and lengthen your torso to your right by keeping the right side of the torso aligned with your right frontal thigh. Bend at the crease of your right hip and not at your waist by keeping both sides of the torso equally lengthening. Tuck the pubic bone slightly in, while the left hip slightly moves forward, exhale, engage abdominals and lower your right arm down above knee, on shin, block or to the floor. Press in to the outer edge of your left leg to anchor yourself. Open your shoulders by rotating your ribcage a little to the left. Keep your palms forward. Feel a line from arm to arm, from shoulder to shoulder. Look up toward your left hand; keep your neck comfortable and in line with the rest of your spine. Imagine that you can fit your body in a narrow space such as between two parallel panels. Breathe for 2-3 breaths.

Tip: *Imagine you are standing against the wall with your shoulders touching the wall.*

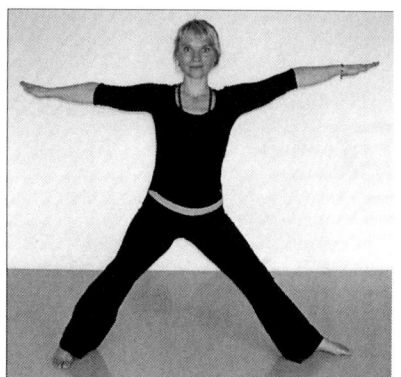

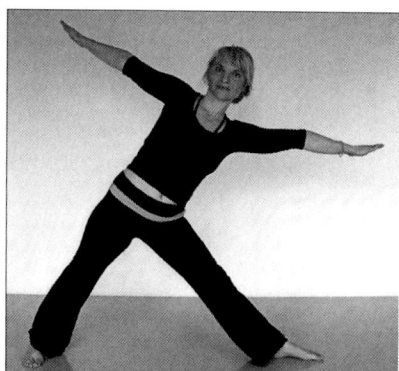

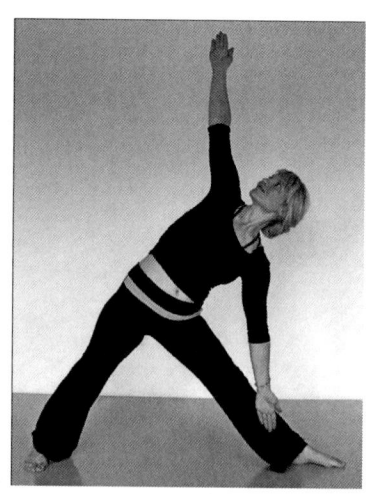

7. Inhale, push the floor away with your feet to come up out of the Triangle pose.

8. Flow into Side Angle Bend. Bend your right knee and open your arms out to the sides with the palms facing up. Inhale and lengthen your torso over your right thigh, exhale and place your right forearm above the knee. Simultaneously, bring your left arm over to the right. Now your left palm will be facing down. Rotate your left hip slightly forward, with your torso and ribcage toward the back wall. Dip your groin down, until your right frontal thigh is parallel to the ground or a little higher. Keep your left leg firm and feel a long line running from the outer edge of the left foot to your fingertips. Look upward to the upper arm bone.

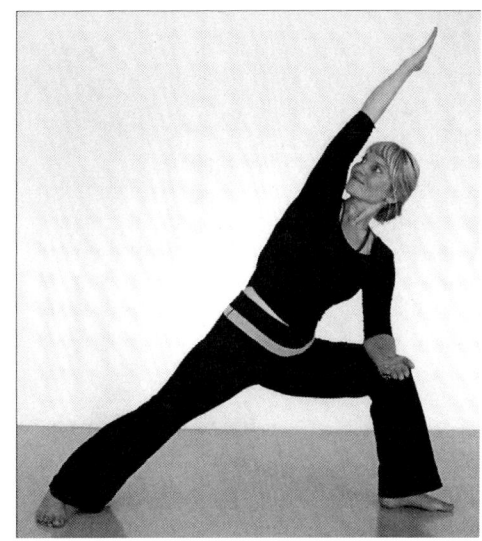

Advanced modification for Side Angle Bend: Hold your ankle or place your hand on the inside of your shinbone. For even more intense pose, place your hand on the ground.

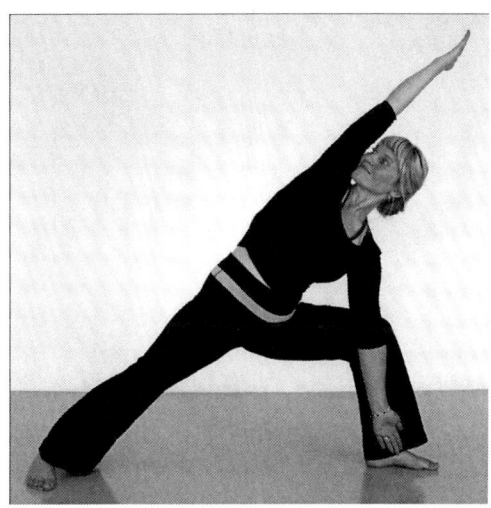

Modifications for tight shoulders:
You can lower your hands on your hips to rest. Keep hand around the small of your back or bend your elbow to open the top of the shoulder.

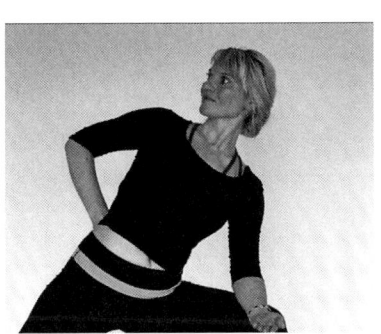
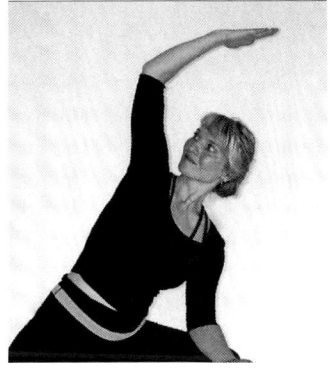

The Heart's Way to Happiness and Health

9. Inhale, press with your feet to come out of the Side Angle Bend. Exhale and lower your arms. Inhale and rotate your hips and torso forward while lifting arms up to the sky to come back to Warrior I. Repeat sequence points four through eight, 3-5 times.

10. Come back to Five Pointed Star, bring your hands to the heart and breathe. Repeat the sequence to the other side 3-5 times.

11. Come back to Five Pointed Star and walk or jump your feet together, into Prayer position. Bring your palms together, breathe and feel.

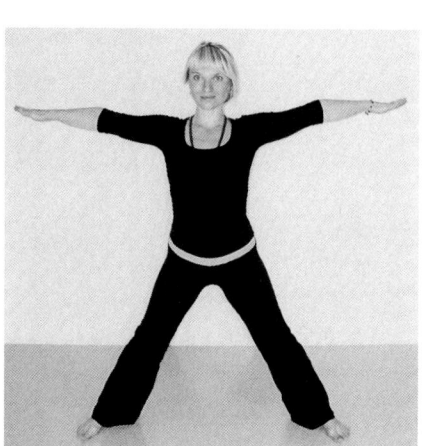
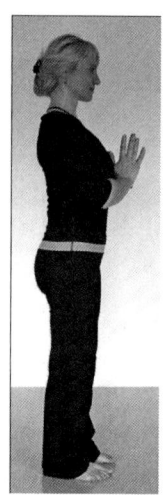

Special Notes: *Keep connection to the ground through your feet in all warrior poses.*

♦ Tree Pose

Purpose: Strengthens standing leg, releases hip flexor muscles in the lifted leg, improves balance and focus.

Sequence:
1. Stand in the mountain pose. Spread and lengthen your toes, root into the ground like a tree through your whole foot.
2. Place right hand on the hip, take hold of your left ankle with your left hand and place your foot on the right inner upper thigh. Keep your pelvis forward but rotate your left knee out to the left. Standing leg is straight but not locked. Keep your abdominals active, lengthen your waist and lift upward through the crown of your head. Feel that your hair is like roots, rooting to the sky.

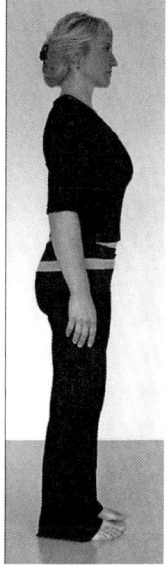
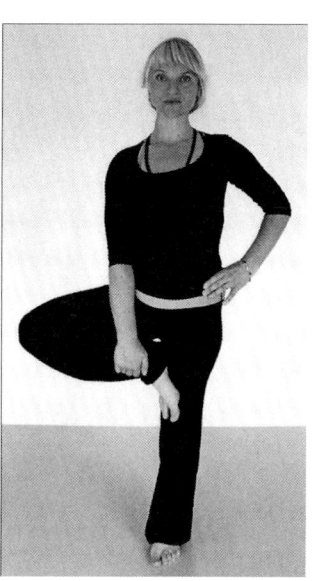

3. Bring your palms together at your heart. Steady your gaze ahead and focus your mind. Slowly bring your arms above your head with elbows bent or straight. Hands together or apart. Hold for 1-2 minutes.

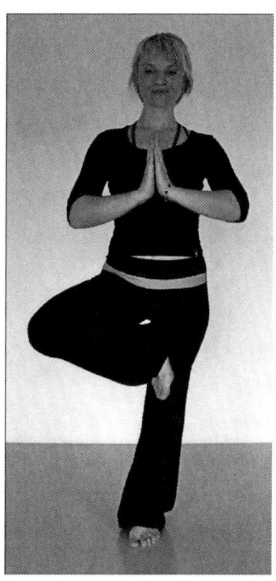
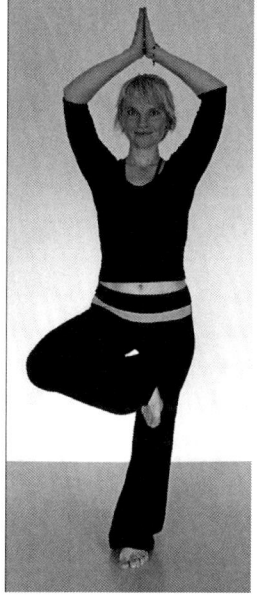

4. Set your foot to the ground, shake your right leg to relax your ankle and leg.

5. Repeat on the other side.

Beginner's modifications:
One foot on top of the other foot or foot below knee. Stand with your back against the wall.

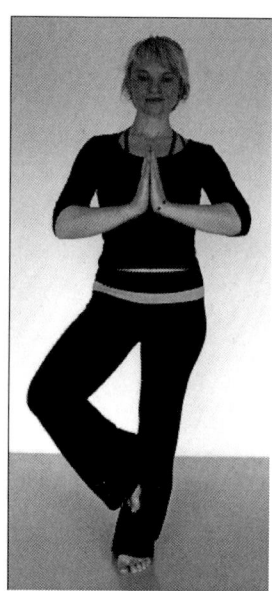

Advanced modification:
Close your eyes.

♦ High Lunge and Crescent Moon Lunge

Purpose: Strengthens legs, core, arms and feet. Improves balance.

Sequence:
1. Inhale and sweep your arms upwards to the Standing Back Bend.
2. Exhale, expand chest, reach arm behind you, hinge at the front of your hips and Forward Bend. Abdominals active.

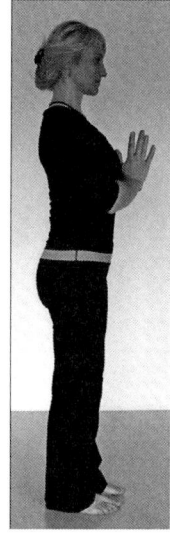
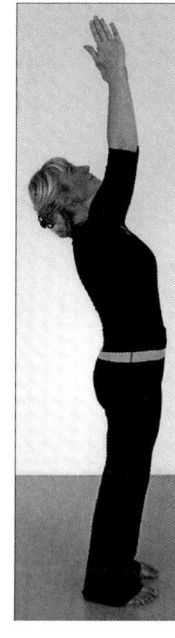

Tip: If it is difficult to touch the ground, start the sequence by placing yoga blocks at the sides of your feet.

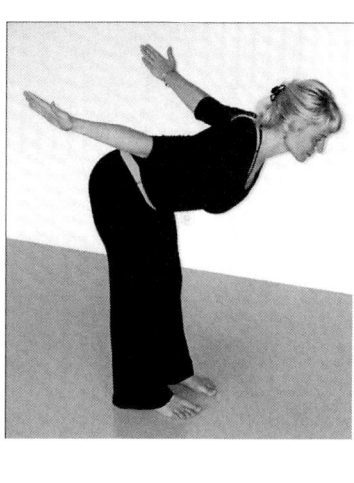
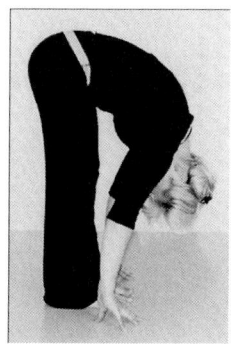

3. Inhale, bend you knees and lengthen your spine from your hips into Spine Extended Forward Bend. Exhale. Step your right foot back into High Lunge and pause for 4-7 breaths.

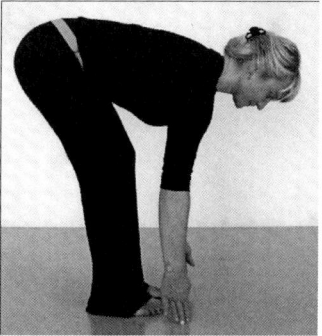
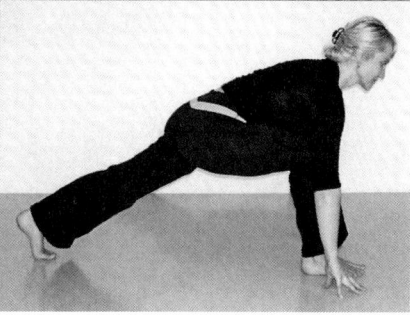

Special Notes for High Lunge: *Keep feet spaced as if they are on railroad tracks and not in line with each other. Feel the connection between your inner thighs. Let your groin stretch by bringing your right upper thigh toward the floor until it is parallel with the ground, if comfortable. Firm your left upper thigh muscles, keeping the knee straight. Draw your left heel back toward the floor. You can have blocks under your hands to help you reach the ground.*

4. Inhale, keep your legs and core strong as you lift your arms up to Crescent Moon Lunge. Hold pose for 4-9 breaths.

Special Notes: Face front knee in the same direction as your foot with knee over your ankle. Do not let the knee push out over your toes. Balance yourself on the ball of your back foot while keeping your back leg strong. Arms straight up, with palms facing. Chest expanded, shoulders broad yet relaxed. Both hips facing forward and pelvis level. Tuck your pubic bone slightly in to lengthen the lower back, activate your abdominals and lift your spine up.

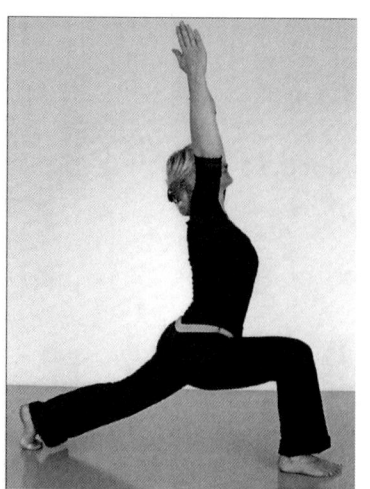

Beginner's modifications for Crescent Moon Lunge:
Keep your hands above the knee to help you with your balance.

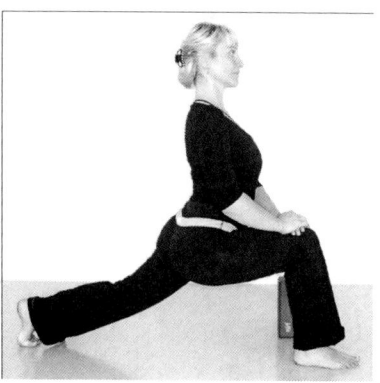

Or skip Lunge sequence and come standing close to the wall. Hold the wall or a chair for balance. Step small step back and reduce the bending in your knees until your legs get stronger.

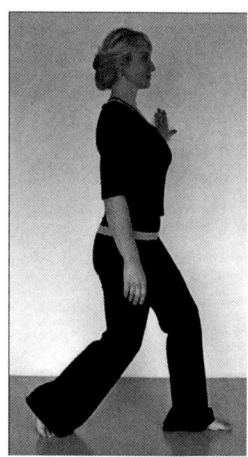
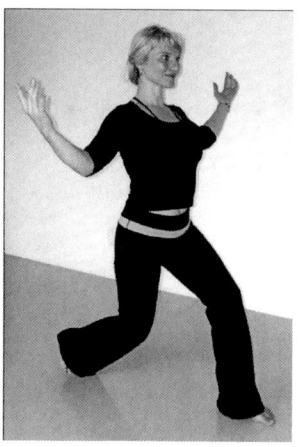

The Heart's Way to Happiness and Health

Advanced variation Lunge with Twist:
While still in the Crescent Moon Lunge, lower your arms and bring your palms together. Inhale, lengthen your spine, exhale, and twist your torso to the right, toward the leg that is in front. Bring your left elbow to the outside of your leg. Press the upper part of your left arm on the outside of your right leg; with your leg resist the arm. Stay in the pose for 3 breaths.

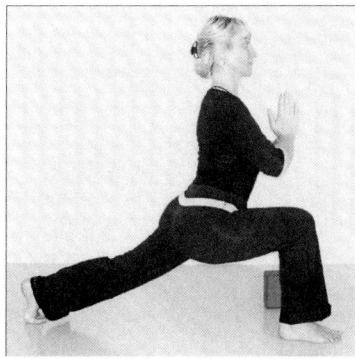 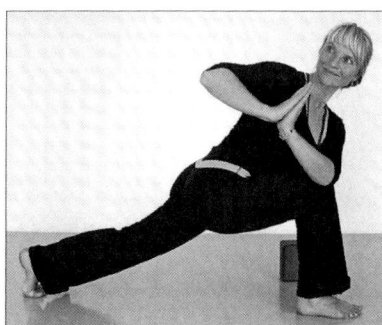

5. Lower arms down to the ground. Step your left foot back to the Downward Facing Dog. Swing your right leg forward and repeat the Crescent Lunge on the other side.

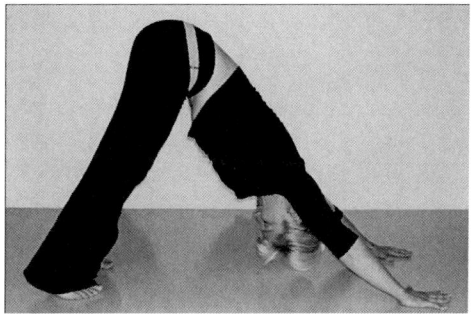

The Heart's Way to Happiness and Health

♦ Garland Pose and Peasant's Squat

Purpose: Improves hip and lower back flexibility.

Caution: Skip points, two through four if you have knee or hip problems. Instead, do beginner's modification.

Sequence:
1. From Downward Facing Dog lower your knees to the ground.

2. Shift your hips on the heels and lift knees off the ground to balance on the balls of your feet. Keep your knees and feet parallel. Lift the crown of your head straight up to the sky. Pause here for 4-9 breaths. Try to lower your heels to the ground and extend arms to the front into the Garland Pose.

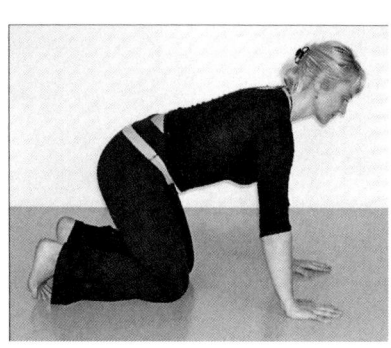 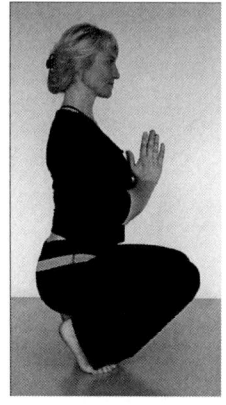 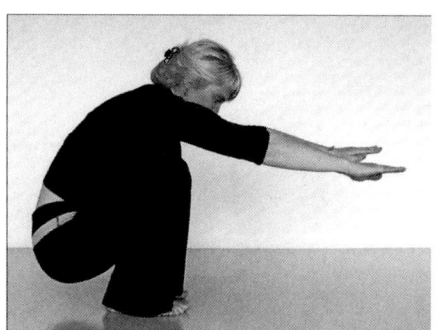

3. Now, open your legs a little wider than your hips, set your feet flat on the ground, rotate your legs outward and squat. Place your elbows on the inside of your legs. Bring your palms together and center your gaze. Straighten your spin, press upper arms into your legs and legs into your arms. Stay in the Pheasant's Squat for 3-5 breaths.

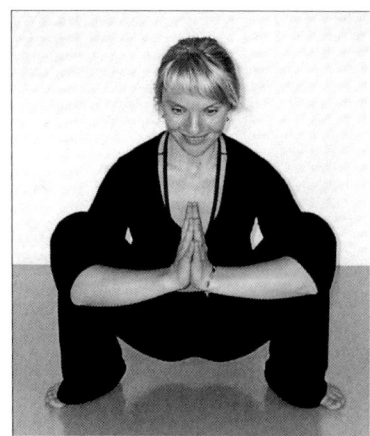

4. Extend arms to the front and bring your hips all away down to the ground, bring knees together, lift feet off the ground and hold hands under your knees, engage abdominals, balance on the sit bones and slowly roll yourself down to the ground to lie down on your back.

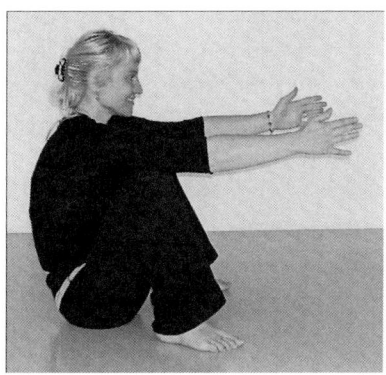
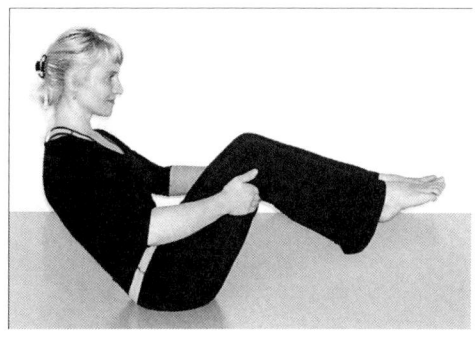

Beginners' modification:
Skip Garland pose and Peasant's squat and instead loosen up your hips in this manner. Once you are on your knees, lie down on your back. Bring knees to chest and separate your knees apart, feel stretch in your inner thighs. Hold for 3-5 breaths and then begin to circle your legs inside of your hip sockets. Circle legs in the hip sockets with legs alternately apart and together, apart and together. Repeat 5 times one way and 5 times the other way. This massages your hips and lubricates the joints. Bring your knees together and lower your feet to the ground.

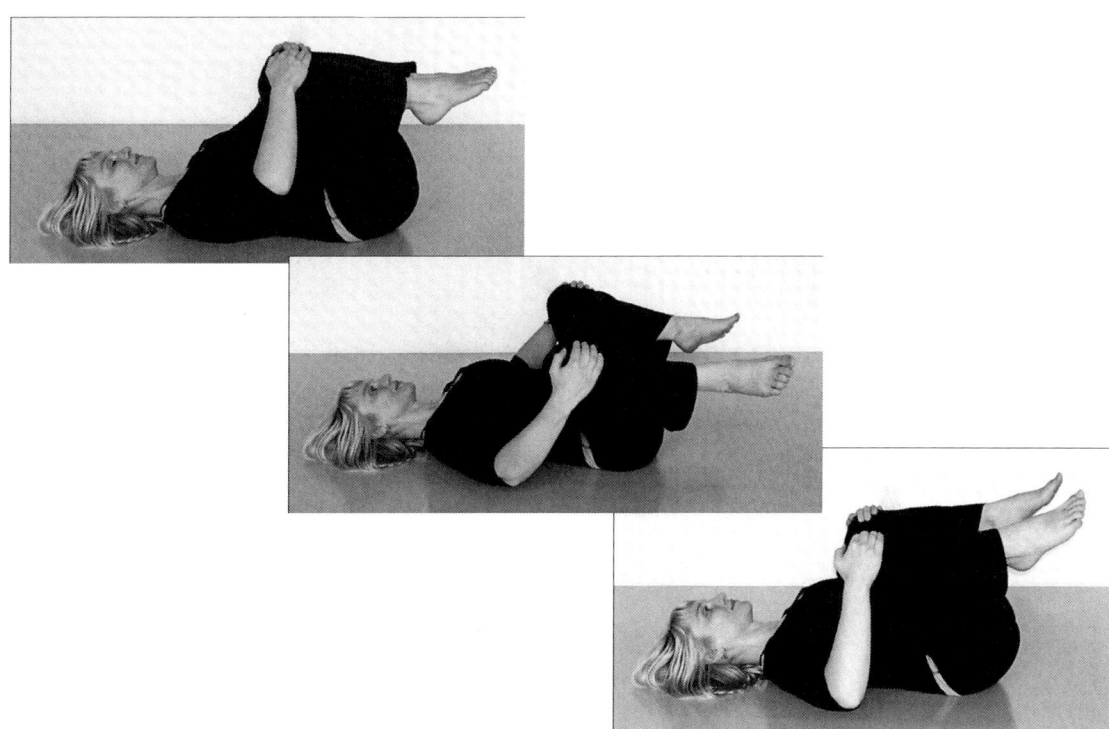

The Heart's Way to Happiness and Health

♦ Boat

Purpose: Strengthens abdominals and hip flexors.

Sequence:
1. Lying on the back. Stabilize your shoulder blades, inhale and lift your arms up to the ceiling, exhale, print your lower back to the floor, zip in the belly as if you are wearing tight pair of jeans, to keep your lower back supported with your abdominals and lift one leg at a time into the Table Top position. Keep your chest open, shoulders broad and back of the neck neutral, slight space under the back of the neck, eyes straight up to the ceiling.

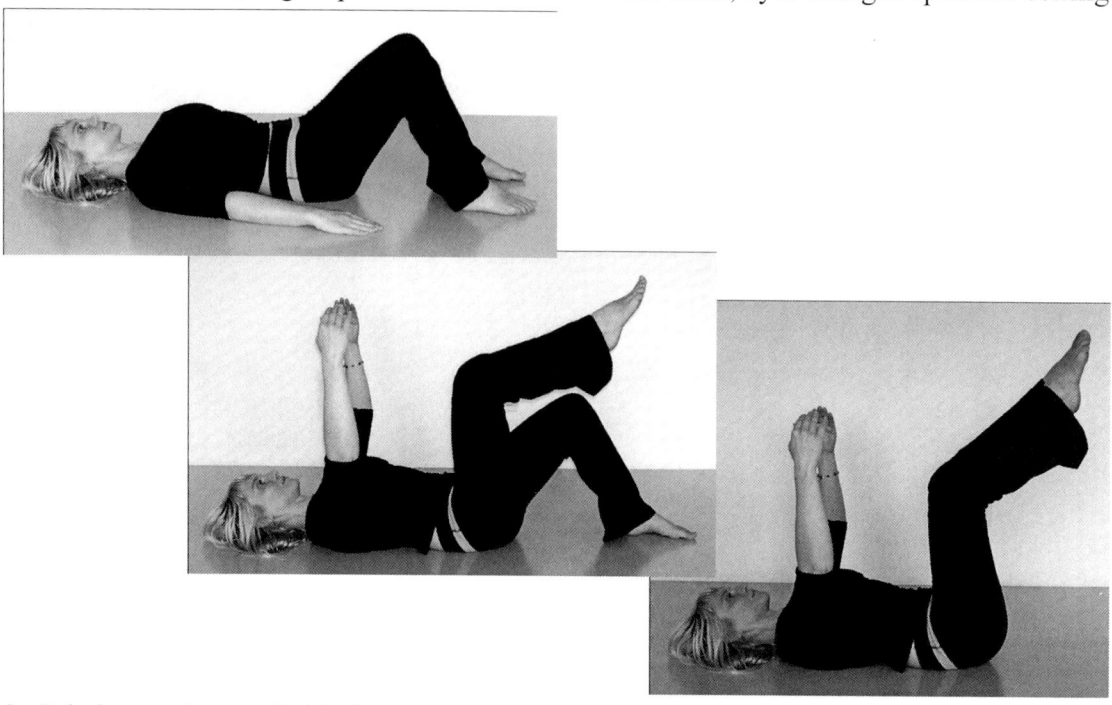

2. Inhale, reach arms behind you.
3. Exhale and lift your head and upper back off the ground. Keep exhaling, hollow your tummy even more and squeeze your inner thighs.

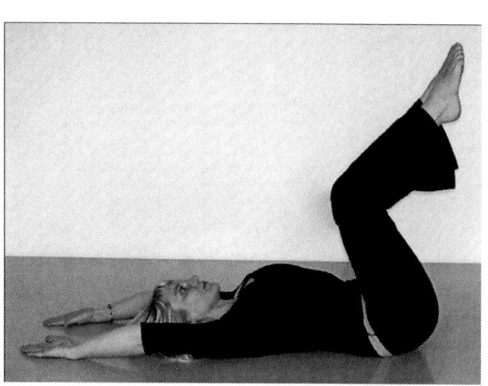
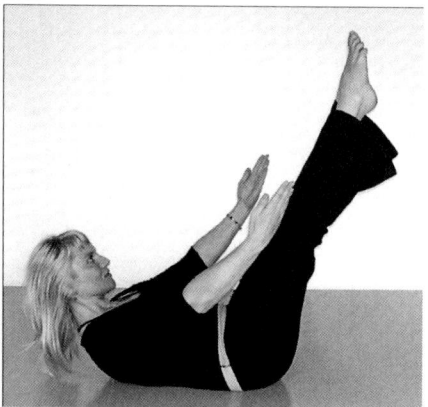

4. Lower your head down to the mat. Inhale, reach arms behind you, and repeat 8-15 times.

Awareness: *Is this comfortable for your neck? You can keep your head on the floor and strengthen your core by lowering straight legs down, hover them above the floor and lift legs back up to the ceiling.*

Special Notes: *It is very important to exhale when you curl up in all abdominal exercises. In all abdominal exercises exhale through your mouth as if you are blowing a candle in front of you and inhale through your nose. If you hold the breath, you are actually deactivating your abdominal muscles. Make sure you inhale into the lower part of your ribcage and not into your abdomen. This will keep your abdomen working and not relaxing.*

Caution: Discontinue any exercise, if it hurts your neck or back.

Advanced modification:
Slowly peel your spine off the floor. As you are coming up, keep your lower back gently rounding. When you are at the top of balance, straighten your spine. And once again, as you lower your spine back down to the ground, begin to round your lower back. Keep your abdominals engaged throughout the exercise.

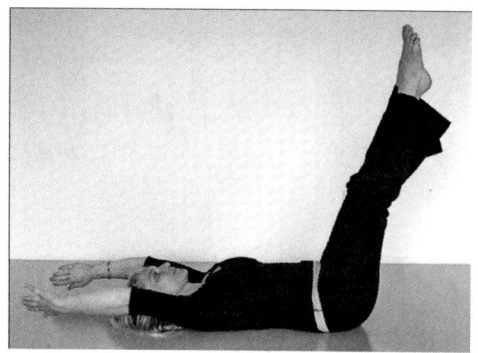

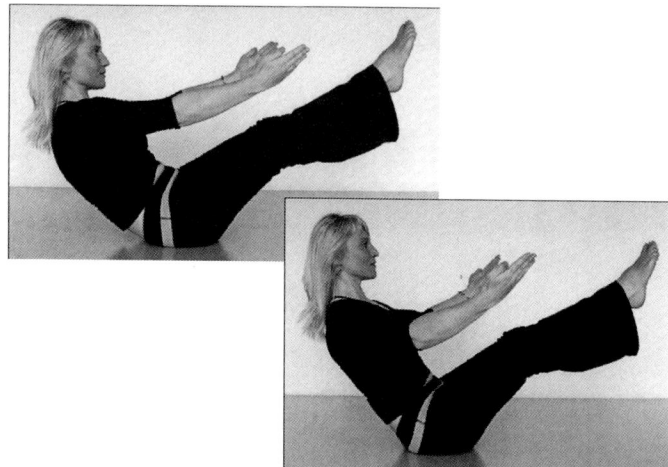

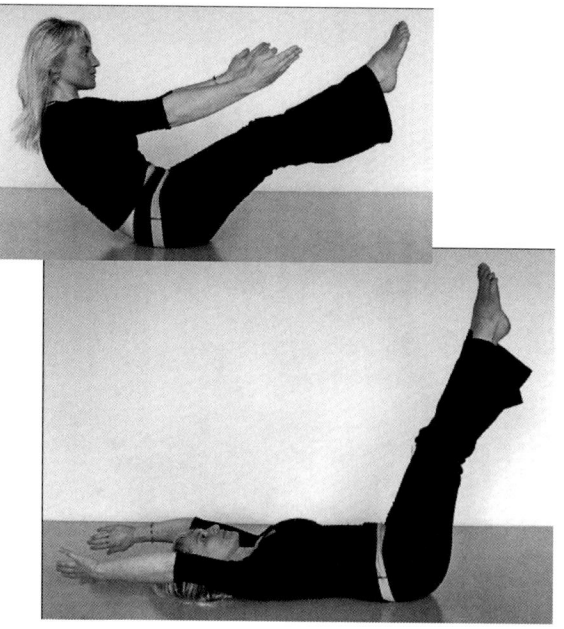

♦ <u>Bicycle</u>

Purpose: Strengthens abdominals.

Sequence:
1. Start in the Table Top position with hands under your head. Inhale and tuck your chin slightly in toward the chest to lengthen the back of the neck

2. Exhale, engage abdominals; lift your head and upper back off the ground.

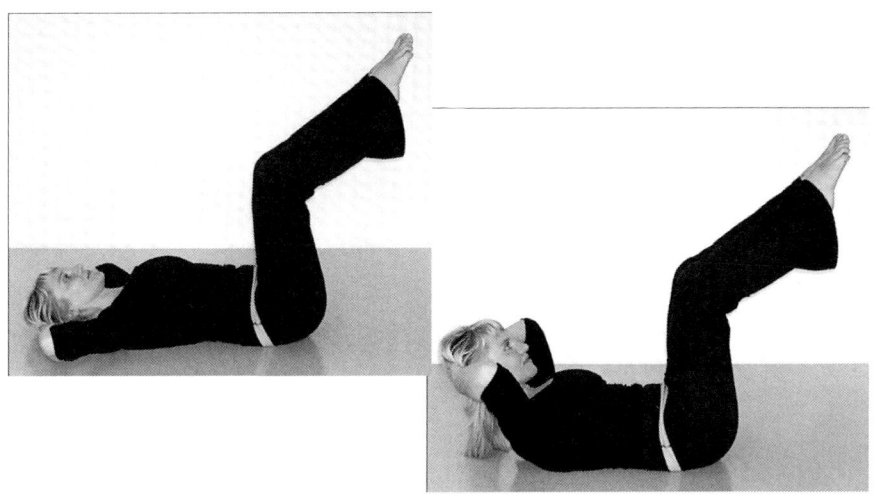

3. Partially inhale and pause. Fully inhaling will relax your abdominals. You want to keep them engaged throughout the exercise.
4. Exhale and lift your left shoulder blade more off the ground as you rotate ribcage to the right.

5. Inhale, come back to the center and keep both shoulder blades lifting off the ground.
6. Exhale, rotate your ribcage to the left as you lift your right shoulder blade off the ground. Keep alternating sides.

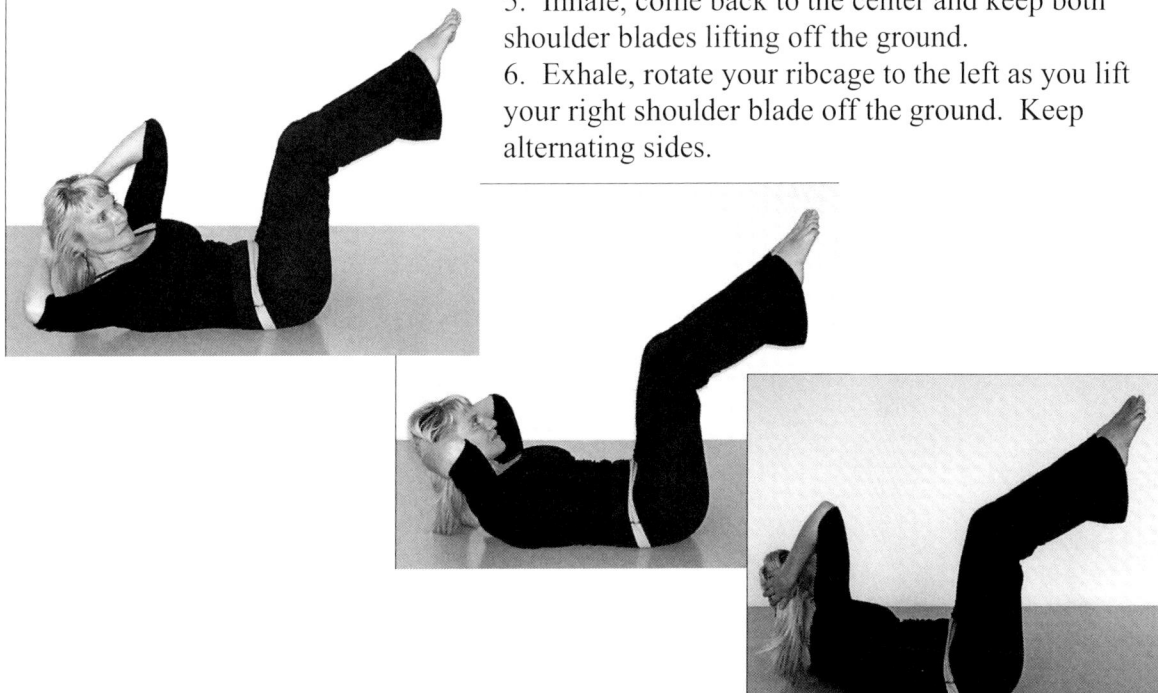

7. Repeat 1-3 sets of 8-15 repetitions to each side.

The Heart's Way to Happiness and Health

Special Notes: *Keep your elbows open, this will help to keep shoulders and neck relaxed. Hips and lower back stable. Remember to exhale through your mouth and inhale through your nose.*

Beginner's modification:

Start with both feet on the ground. Lift your right leg as you bring the left elbow toward the knee. Lower your right foot and keep alternating the sides.

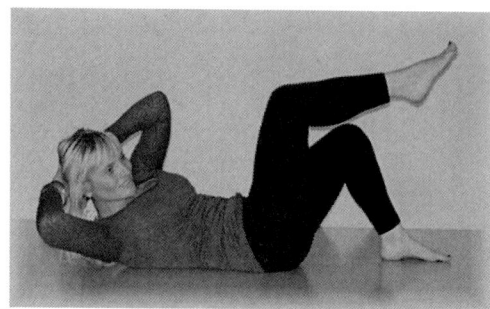

Advanced modification:

Add leg movement to this exercise. Bring right elbow to the left knee and extend the right leg by firming your thigh muscles. Now switch sides, bring your left elbow to the right knee and extend left leg. Keep your pelvis and lower back stable. Imagine you have springs pushing with your feet. As you straighten the leg, push against the resistance of the imaginary spring. This will help to keep your upper thigh firm and pelvis stable.

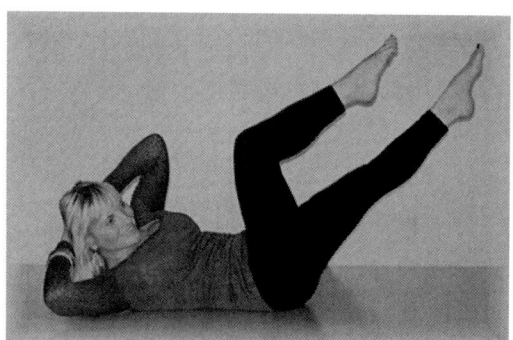

♦ Bridge

Purpose: Strengthens buttocks, legs and lower back.

Sequence:

1. Lying on your back, bend the knees and place a block or a folded towel between your inner thighs. Keep feet parallel and hip distance apart. Connect to the ground with your whole foot (your big toe, small toe and your heel). Arms at your sides and front of the shoulders open.

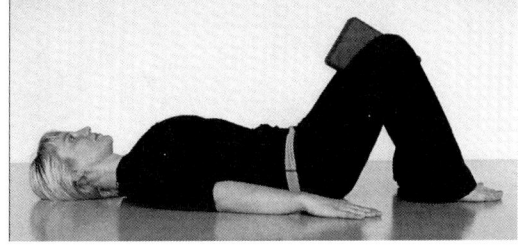

2. Inhale and lift your hips off the floor, exhale and lower. Repeat 10-20 times.

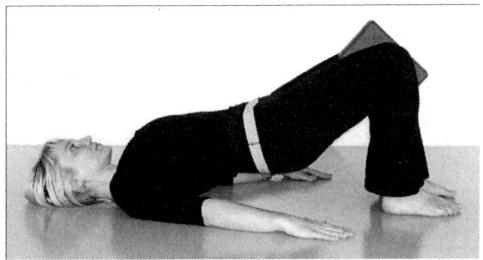

Special Notes: *Tuck the pubic bone slightly in, lengthen your tailbone and pubic bone toward the knees. Keep your sternum in line with your pubic bone for more neutral alignment. Make sure your neck is long and there is a slight space between your chin and your chest.*

3. Now, again lift your hips off the ground but this time instead of lowering your hips down to the floor, lower them only a few inches down and lift them back up. Lower a few inches and lift 10-20 times.

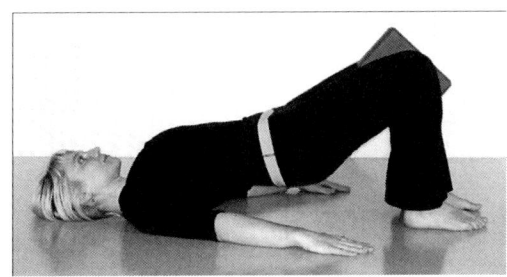
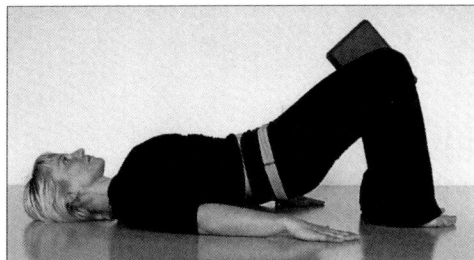

The Heart's Way to Happiness and Health

4. Inhale, and on your next exhale lower hips down to the ground, set block or towel aside and hug the knees to your chest. Breathe.

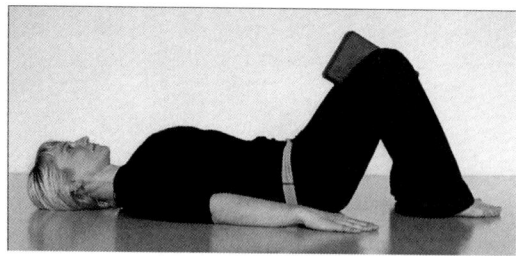

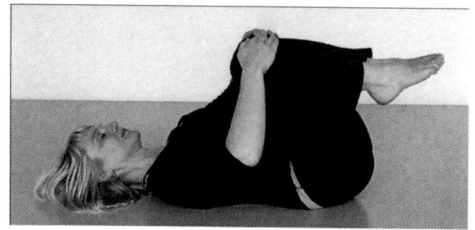

♦ <u>Side Leg Lifts and Inner Thigh Lifts</u>

Purpose: Tones thighs and buttocks.

Sequence:
1. Lying on your side, keep spine elongated, head in line with your hips. Place bottom arm under the head. Bend your bottom leg for stability and straighten your top leg. Keep your top hip stacked on top of the bottom hip. Stack shoulder on top of the shoulder. Support your balance with your top hand in front of your ribcage.

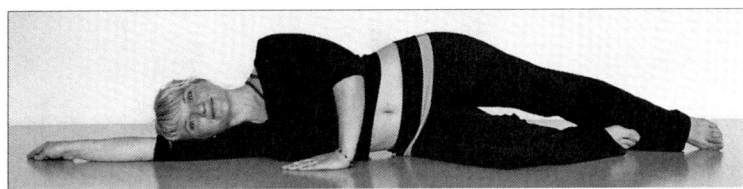

2. Using the buttock, inhale and leading with a heel, lift your top leg up, a little higher than your hip, exhale and lower your leg all the way down. Repeat 10-20 times.

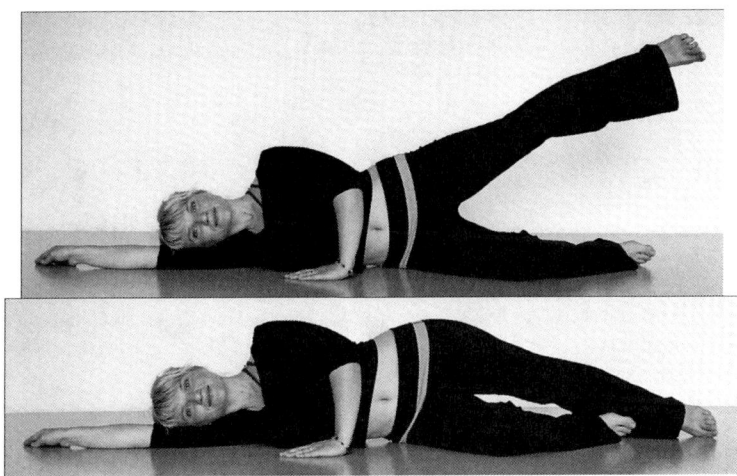

3. This time lower your top leg half way down, about at the level of your hip. Lift the leg up again and repeat 10-20 times.

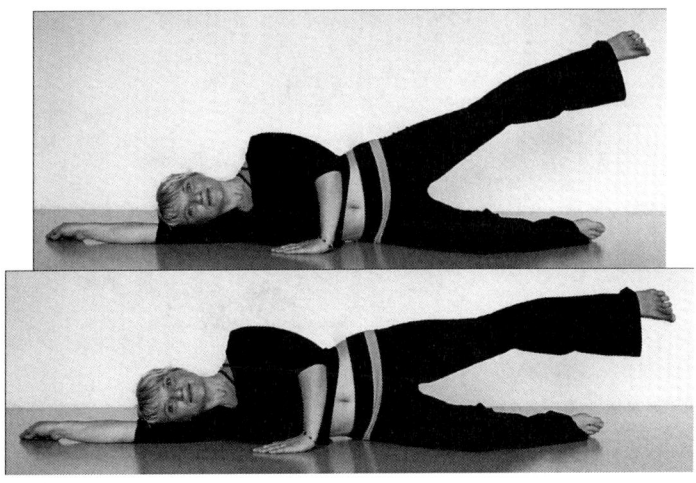

4. Bend your top knee and place it on the ground in front of your bottom leg. Point toes and lift your bottom leg up using your inner thigh muscles. Lower leg down an inch or so off the ground. Repeat, lifting and lowering your leg 10 times. Now, flex your ankle and repeat leg lifts, 10 times. On the last repetition hold leg up and circle it above the ground 10 times one way with ankle flexed and 10 time the other way with toes pointing.

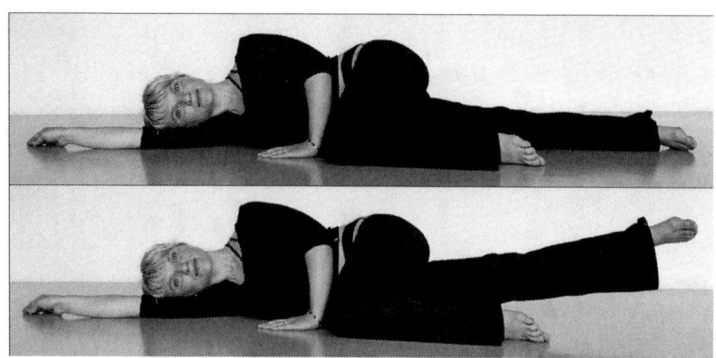

5. Straighten and firm your legs. Inhale and lift both legs off the floor at your hips, not at your waist. Squeeze your legs together, hold for 1 second, exhale and slowly lower legs down. Repeat 10-20 times.

Tip: Place a large sponge for washing cars under your bottom hip to relieve pressure between bottom hip and floor.

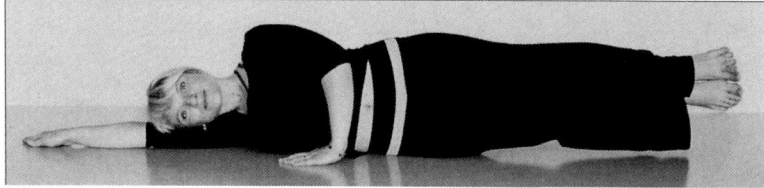

Advanced modification:
Place your top hand on top of your leg. Inhale and press your bottom arm into the ground. Exhale, squeeze your inner thighs together. Firm your legs, use your waist muscles to lift the bottom side of your ribcage and your legs off the floor. Inhale, look and reach fingertips toward your feet. Exhale and lower.

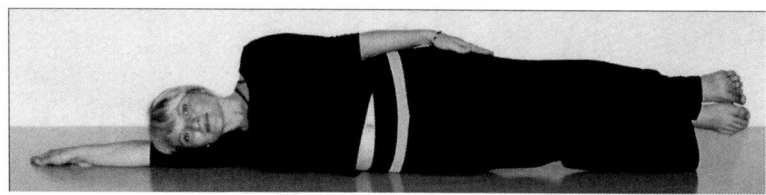

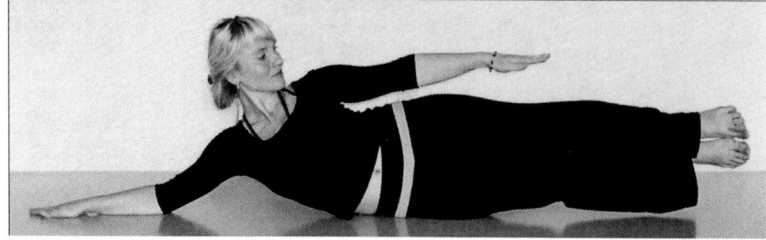

6. Roll on the other side and repeat the sequence.

♦ <u>Swimming</u>

Purpose: Lengthens the spine, strengthens abdominals, arms, back, buttocks and legs.

Sequence:
1. Lie on your abdomen and extend the arms in front of you. Keep your forehead on the mat. Legs, hip distance apart.

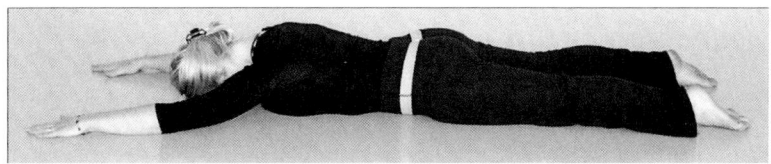

2. Inhale and lift your right arm and left leg off the floor. Lift your face and chest also.

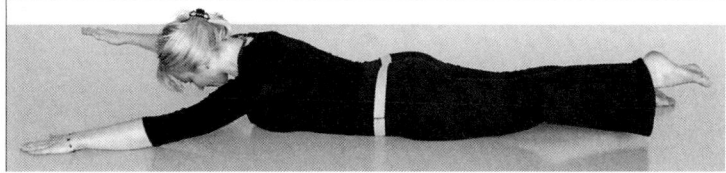

3. Exhale, lower.
4. Inhale, lift left arm and right leg. Exhale, lower.
5. Keep alternating the sides for 8-15 repetitions on each leg.

Special Notes: *Keep your face parallel to the ground and shoulders away from your ears. Activate your abdominals and buttock muscles to lift your leg. Your hips should both be level and face the ground throughout the exercise. Your box, that is from shoulder to shoulder, hip to hip, should be very stable.*

Awareness: *Can you feel the muscles at the bottom tip of your scapula and on the sides of your ribcage? These muscles stabilize your shoulder blades and keep them broad across your back.*

Beginner's modification:
1. Keep your face on the ground to relax your neck.

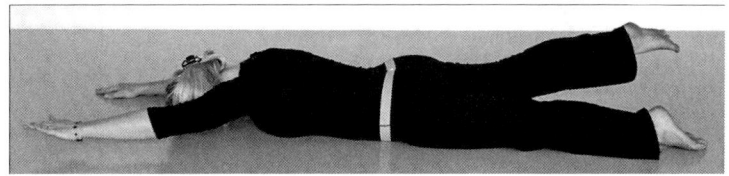

2. If it is too much for your back, place hands under the forehead and lift one leg. Keep alternating your legs.

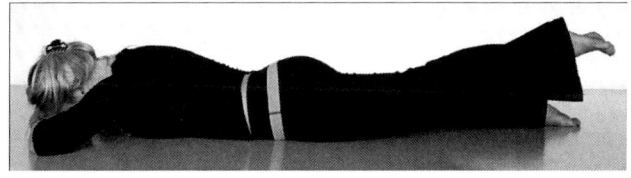

Advanced modification:
1. Inhale and lift both arms and legs off the ground simultaneously

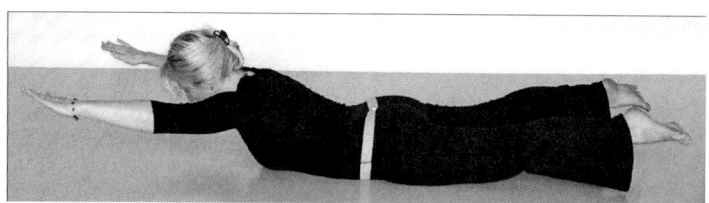

2. Move your opposite arm and leg, keep switching them above the ground. You can also do this movement at a faster pace. Imagine you are splashing water with your arms and legs. Repeat for 30 seconds to 1 minute, 1-3 sets.

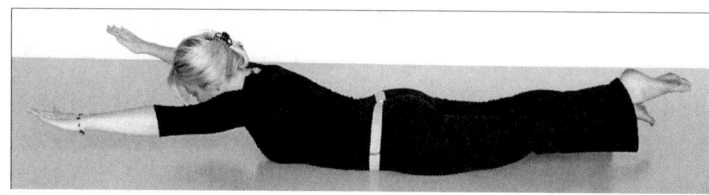

3. Inhale, pause and lengthen through your arms and legs in the air.

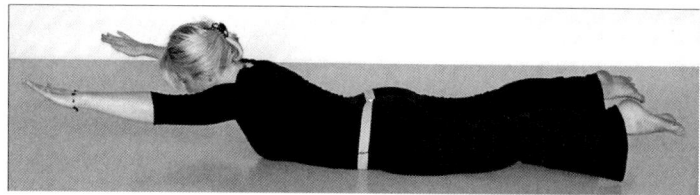

4. Exhale and lower your extremities down to finish the exercise.

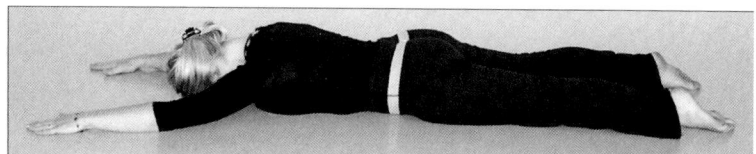

◆ <u>Locust</u>

Purpose: Strengthens abdominals, back, buttocks and legs. Opens chest and shoulders.

Sequence:

1. Lie on your abdomen and bring arms to the sides of your legs. Palms facing up. Keep your forehead on the mat. Legs, hip distance apart.

2. Press the tops of your feet into the ground to engage your legs. Activate your abdominals, inhale and lift your face and chest. Lift your arms. Expand chest and keep your shoulder blades wide across your back. Lift your legs off the ground or keep them on the ground for the lower back comfort.

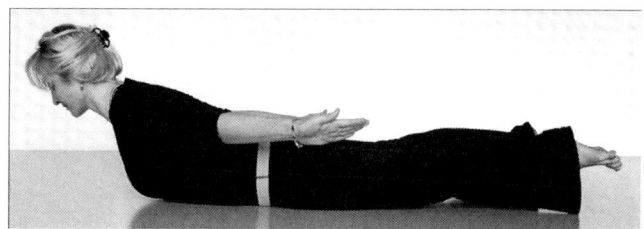

3. Exhale and lower. You can turn your head to one side and rest for a few seconds.

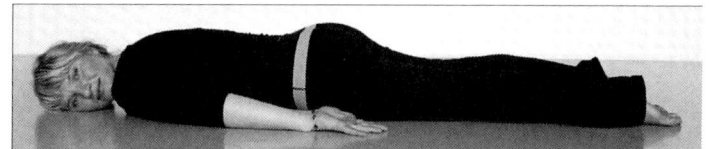

4. Repeat 4 times.

5. On the last one, hold the pose for 3-5 breaths.

Advanced modification:
On the last repetition, clasp your hands behind your back, bring your shoulder blades gently together. Lift and reach your knuckles comfortably toward your feet and hold for 3-5 breath cycles.

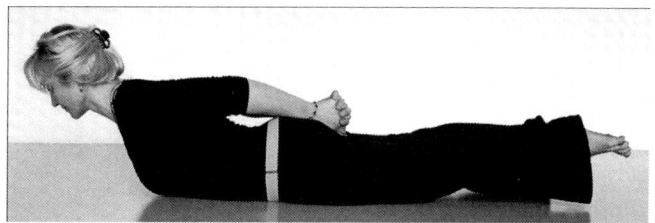

Awareness: *Any time your back is too tired, rest in the child's pose.*

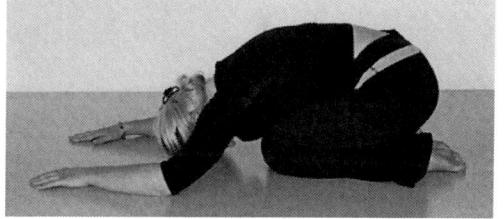

The Heart's Way to Happiness and Health

♦ Hip Opener

Purpose: Stretches buttocks and opens hips.

Sequence:

1. Lie on your back with knees bent. Place your right ankle above your left knee.

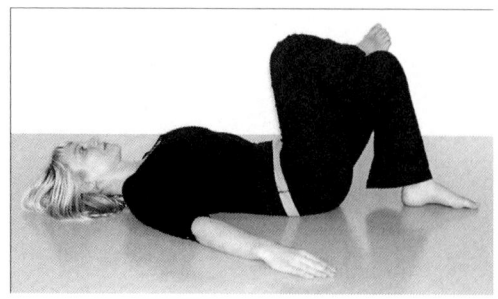

2. Lift your left foot off the ground. Place right hand between the legs and left hand on the outside of the left leg to interlace your fingers around the back of your left leg. Rotate your right hip toward the wall in front of you. Feel the stretch in the right buttock area. Hold for 1-2 minutes.

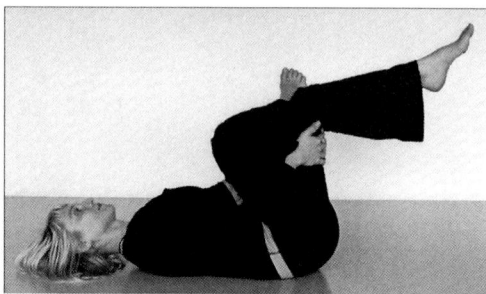

3. Lower foot to the ground and repeat on the other side.

Beginner's modification:

If it is too difficult to hold the back of the leg with your hands, instead, keep legs straight on the ground, bend right knee to chest and draw it with your hands to the opposite shoulder.

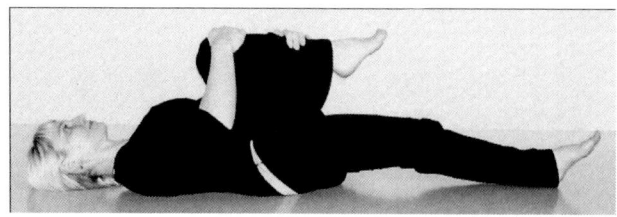

♦ <u>Plow and Shoulder Stand</u>

Purpose: Stretches lower back and hips, promotes circulation, rests feet and legs, opens upper back, promotes restful sleep, stimulates thyroid.

Caution: Skip inversion pose, if you are menstruating, pregnant or have back, neck or shoulder pain, have high blood pressure, eye strain or ear infection.

Sequence:
1. Lying on the back, bend knees and lift legs up to the ceiling. Exhale and use your abdominals to bring your hips off the floor, legs behind you. Simultaneously, bend your elbows, press upper arms into the floor and place hands on your back. Try to bring your elbows in line with shoulders by rolling your shoulders under and bringing your shoulder blades together. Your feet can be above the ground or on the floor behind your head. Flex your ankles and reach through the heels.
Breathe smoothly for 4-9 breaths.

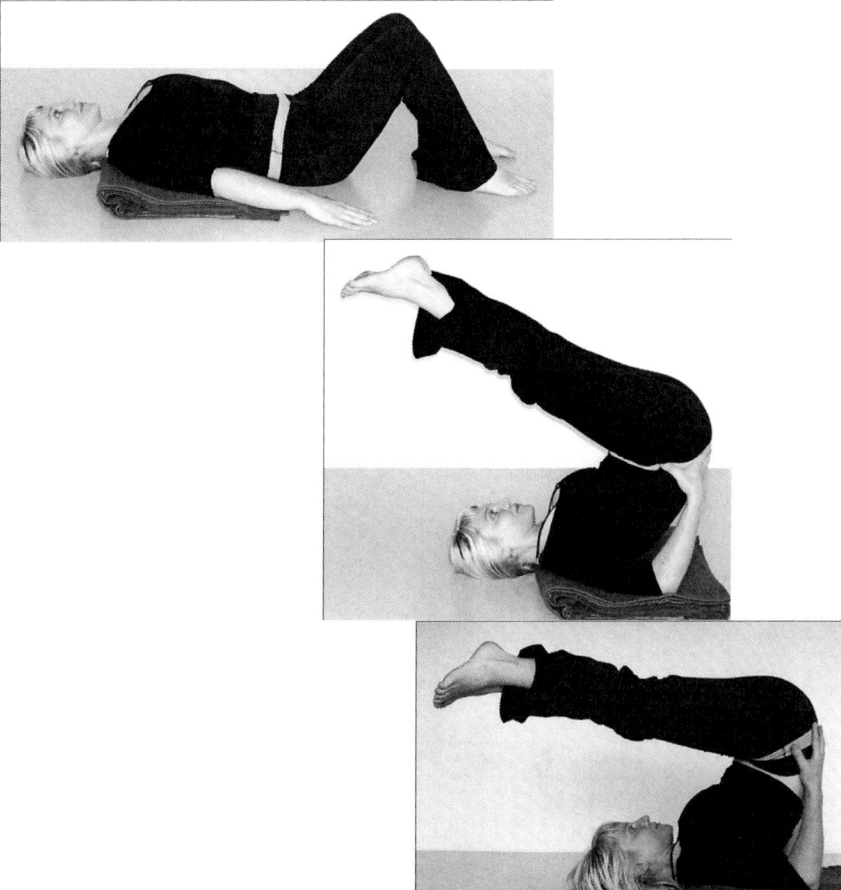

Special Notes: *To protect your neck, make sure you don't look side to side in this pose. Keep your eyes always up to the ceiling.*
You can place the blanket under your upper back, neck off the blanket, to create a little more space between neck and floor, thus, positioning neck in more neutral curves.

The Heart's Way to Happiness and Health

2. Engage abdominals, inhale and slowly lift your legs up to the ceiling, until your toes are in line with your eyes. Lift your hips up until you are balanced on top of your upper back and there is no pressure in the neck. Lengthen through your inner thighs, toes and keep your legs together, abdominals and pelvic floor active. Breathe 4-9 breath cycles.

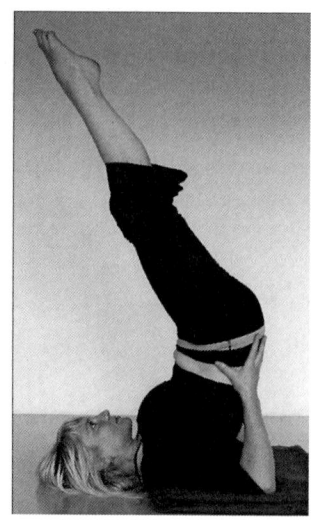

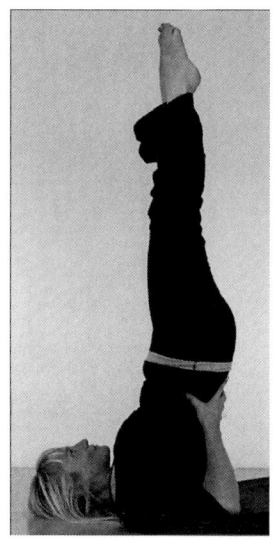

Advanced modification:
Align your thighs with your torso, so that you will be in a straight line.

4. To come out of the pose, lower legs comfortably behind you again, bend your knees and slowly with abdominal control lower your hips down to the ground, assisting with your hands as needed.

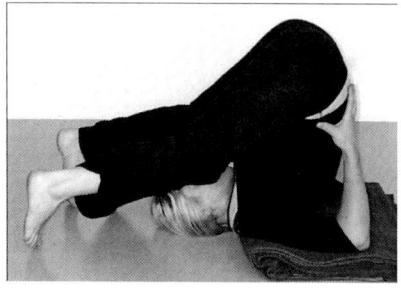
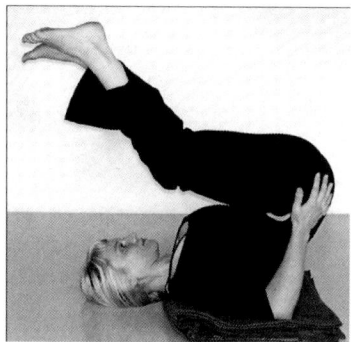

5. Straighten legs on the mat, open arms out at your sides, relax, feel and breathe for a few moments.

Modification Legs-up-the Wall:

Sit sideways, parallel to the wall; simultaneously, as you lift your legs up against the wall, lower and rotate your torso to the ground, so that your hips are even and as close to the wall as possible. Stay in this pose for 5-10 minutes. To come out of this pose, bend your knees, and gently roll on your side.

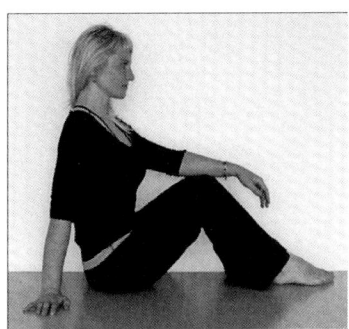

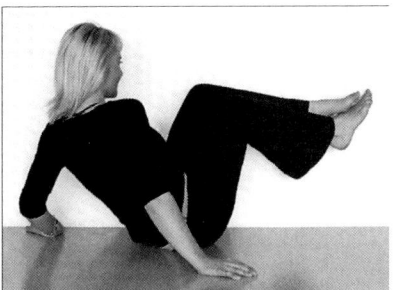

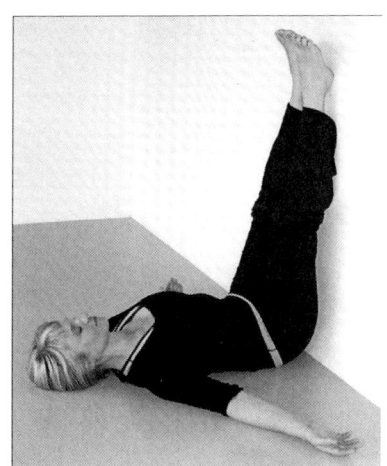

The Heart's Way to Happiness and Health

♦ <u>Cobra Pose</u>

Purpose: Strengthens back and legs. Expands chest and stretches shoulders and abdomen.

Sequence:

1. Begin by lying down on your abdomen. Place hands under your shoulders. Forehead to the ground, back of the neck long, elbows pointing straight back and close to the body. Keep your shoulders away from your ears and upper back wide.

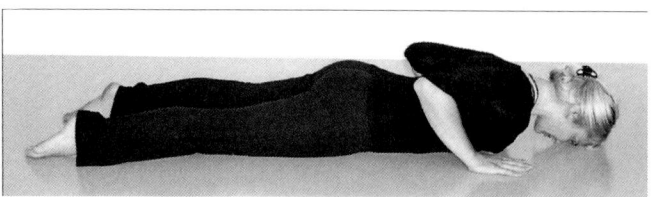

2. Activate your abdominals and firm the legs. As you inhale, imagine you have a marble under your nose, roll the marble with the nose to lift your head, then lift your neck and finally chest. Tuck your pubic bone slightly in to lengthen and protect your lower back. You can stop at the bottom of your ribs or press into your hands and lift your lower ribs off the ground, while keeping hips on the floor. Reach your heart forward, elbows pointing straight back and close to the body to Cobra pose.

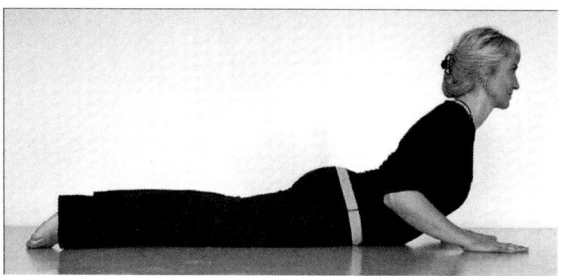

3. Exhale and lower to initial position sequentially: at first ribs, then chest and finally your head. Repeat Cobra pose 3-5 times.

4. After doing all repetition. Pause lying on your abdomen and breath into you lower back and hips for as long as you like.

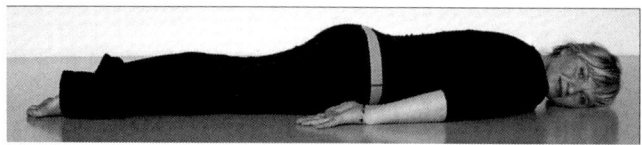

♦ <u>Hip Twist</u>

Purpose: Stretches outer hip, releases pelvis, lower back, opens shoulders and chest.

Sequence:
1. Lying on the ground, outstretch your arms to the sides. Scoot your hips a little to the left.

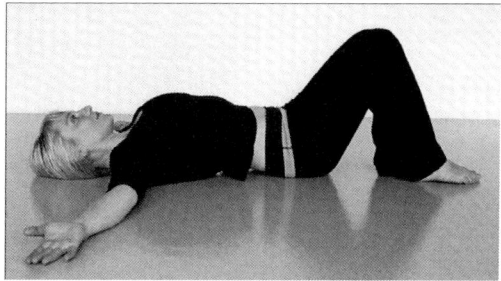

2. Inhale, lift your legs off the ground, exhale and lower your legs to the right. Lift the left side of your hip up to stack it over your right side. Relax neck to the left. Pause in this position for 4-9 breaths.

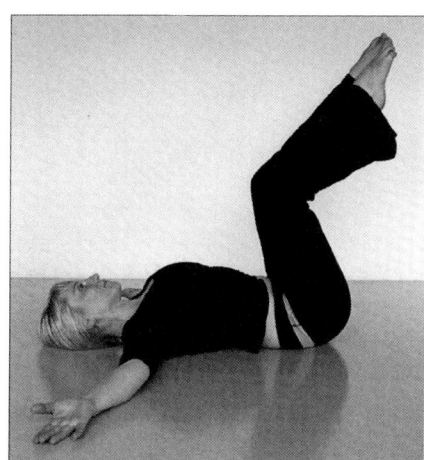
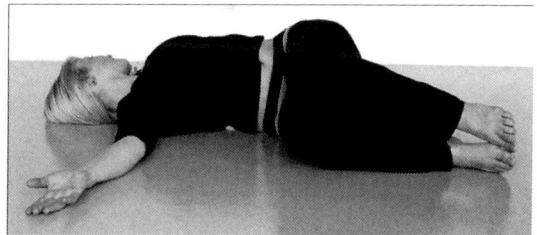

Special Notes: *You can place your right hand on the outside of the left thigh to deepen the stretch in your outer left hip.*

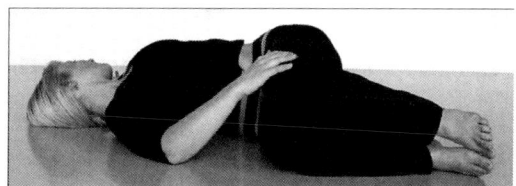

The Heart's Way to Happiness and Health

You can also stretch your left leg straight out to the right.

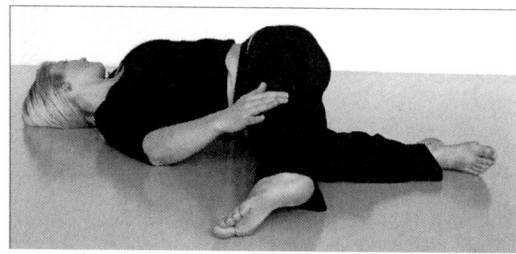

3. If your leg is outstretched, stack your legs together, inhale and use your abdominals to lift the legs back to the center, exhale and lower both feet to the ground. Shift hips a little to the right and repeat the twist by lowering the legs to the left.

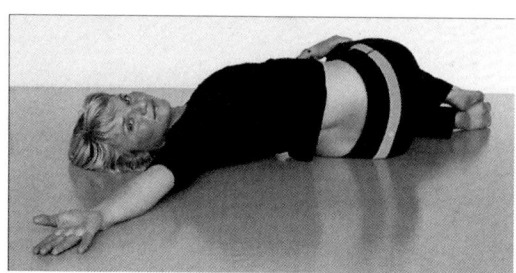

Modification:
Keep the feet on the ground and lower the legs to the right side, while lifting the left side of your hip up. Repeat by lowering your legs side to side a few times.

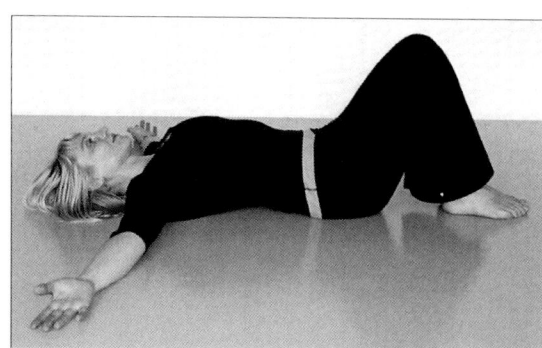

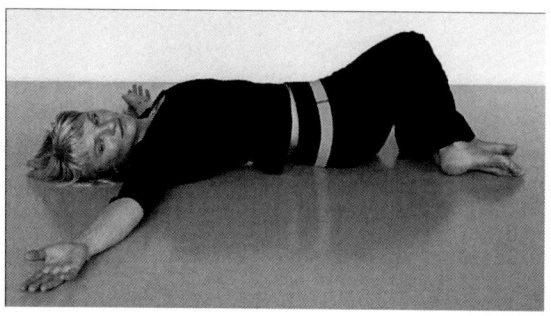

♦ Savasana or Restorative Relaxation

Purpose: Relax completely, renew, restore, let go, and rebalance.

Sequence:
1. Lying on your back, legs completely relaxed, rotated outward at your hips. Arms resting at your sides with palms up and front of your shoulders open.

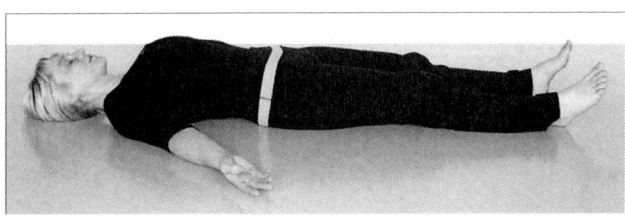

2. Scan your body from toes to crown of your head, allow yourself to completely relax and melt into the ground. If you are feeling tension anywhere, send love to that area, feel how your body responds to the loving care.
3. Allow your organs to soften as well. Feel your heart beat, feel love entering and filling your whole body, radiating through your pores.
4. Now and then feel your belly rise and fall as you are breathing. Do not control, speed up or hold your breath. Let it happen, as if you are watching whole universe breathing through you.
5. Practice Savasana for 5-15 minutes. Try not to drift to sleep. Be conscious and relaxed.

Awareness: Make yourself comfortable. You can use a towel under your head to support your neck, or a rolled blanket under your knees to relax your lower back. If you are cool, cover yourself with a blanket.

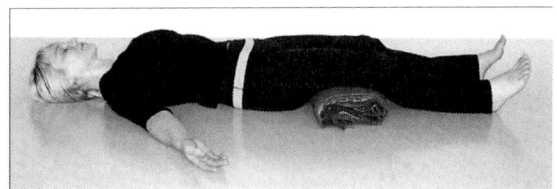

The Heart's Way to Happiness and Health

6. To come up, wiggle fingers and toes, bend your knees and gently roll on your right side to the fetal position. Pause in the fetal position for some time and use your hands to slowly come up to a seated position.

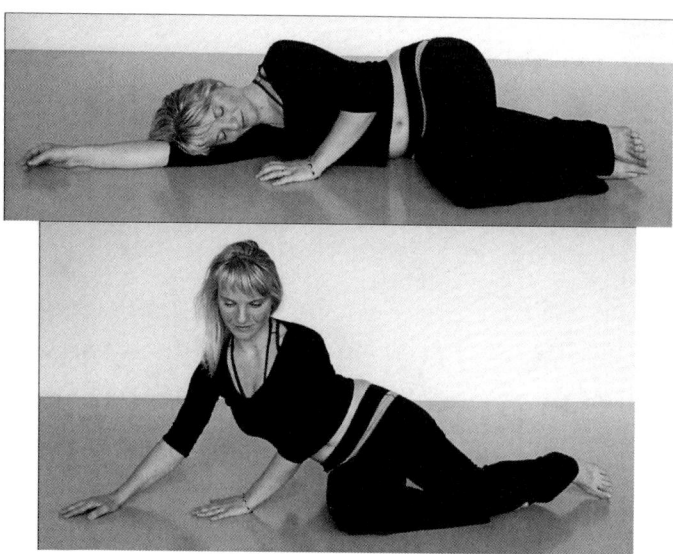

7. Place your hands on the heart and ask yourself a question: if I plant you, what will you grow? You might receive an answer as a thought, image, color or feeling.   Pause.

Bring your palms together at your heart, say to yourself a prayer or affirmation, feel what you are saying with your whole being. Feel the smile in your heart.

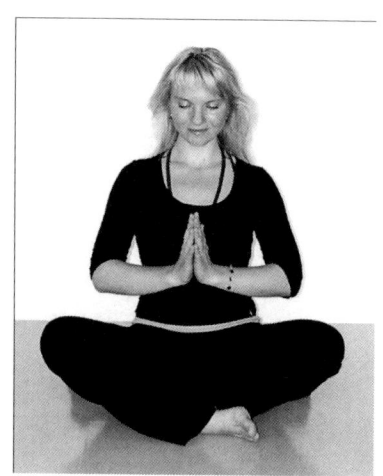

Namaste

(To find out the meaning of "namaste," see CONCLUCION *p. 101)*

Feeling Good in Your Body Tips

- **Practice deep breathing daily.**

    Remember to take deep breaths throughout the day. Mindful breathing will center and calm your mind, increase your energy levels, activate your immune system and improve function of every vital organ.

    Our lymph system is responsible for the production of white blood cells that fight disease-causing pathogens. Unlike the cardiovascular system, the lymphatic system does not have a pump for pumping lymph fluid. The only way to stimulate our lymph system is through deep, correct breathing, laughter and movement. The following exercises help us to retrain ourselves away from shallow upper chest breathing to open diaphragm, lungs and deeper breathing for better health.

    ***Awareness - Belly Breathing:** Assume a good posture. Imagine that your breathing muscles are like a cylinder. The top of the cylinder is your diaphragm, the bottom of the cylinder is your pelvic floor, and the walls of the cylinders are your deep abdominal muscles that run like a corset all around your torso.*

    Begin by exhaling all air out of your lungs through your nose for a count of 5-10, pull the abdominals in and feel you are ringing all air out of your lungs. On your next inhale, feel the top of the cylinder (diaphragm) sliding downward expanding your abdomen, ribcage and chest. Keep your shoulders relaxed. Pause. On your exhale feel your ribcage relax, the walls of the cylinder (your abdominal muscles) pull inward while the bottom of the cylinder (pelvic floor) contract/pull up. Keep breathing deeply for 5-10 minutes.

    ***Special Notes:** Breathe through your nose, keep your pace comfortable, slow down, feel the pauses between the exhalations and inhalations. Make the breathing smooth, deep and at the same time effortless. Be patient as it takes practice to re-learn a natural way of breathing.*

> *derror**Improve your Voice:** Try this experiment; inhale and exhale through your nose.*
>
> *Now hum for 1 minute, be fun, vary your speed and loudness. Don't hum a tune, simply make sounds.*
>
> *Now again inhale through you nose. Do you feel how your nasal passages have cleared and you were able to take in a deeper breath? Singing, humming, making vowel sounds, very loudly and very softly, clears your voice, opens lungs and improves the sound of your voice. So, next time you have a commute why not to practice an aria from your favorite opera or simply shouting and having fun with a variety of sounds will do the trick.*

> *Finding your true voice lesson:*
>
> *Say it very loudly from your abdomen, deep from within your belly:*
> *Aaaaaaaaaaa*
> *Ooooooooooooo*
> *Uuuuuuuuuuuu*
> *Eeeeeeeeeeeeee*
>
> *Try whispering, singing, humming and making a variety of sounds.*

- **Exercise your physical body mindfully.**

  Exercise should be a part of your <u>daily life</u>. If you are a beginner, start with at least 10 minutes of exercise daily. Gradually add time until you build up to 1 hour. Your workouts should be challenging but not to the point of pain. If you are a beginner, you will experience more sore muscles 1-3 days after your workouts; however, to be healthy there is no need to always be sore after each workout. It is more important to be regular with your movement and exercise program than to push yourself hard every time.

  As you exercise, you will feel the burn in your muscles. That's good. But you should learn to differentiate between pain and healthy muscle fatigue. You should reduce the intensity of an exercise or discontinue it, if you are feeling the discomfort and stiffness in your joints. In the right level of workout, you are challenging yourself but you are able to breathe.

  Awareness: *Be in tune with your body, if you are tired then do a lighter, shorter workout, you will be surprised that by the end of the workout you actually will have more energy than when you started. On the other hand, if you feel very energetic, then make your activity more vigorous and challenging!*

> <u>*What type of personality are you?*</u> *If you like variety in your life than vary your exercises to keep you muscles and your mind from getting bored on a regular basis. If you like stability it is ok to stick with one exercise regimen that works for you. Remember that the body, just like mind needs to be stimulated and challenged in different ways. So try adding a few new exercises at least once a month.*

- **Stretch daily.**

  Flexibility will help you to avoid injuries. It is important to maintain a balance between being strong and being flexible.

- **Take short breaks from computer.**

  If you work at the computer, give yourself a break every hour. You are meant to move, form the prehistoric times we have been hunters and gatherers. We are not meant to sit at the computer! Get up from the computer every hour and perform a few stretches, relax your eyes and simply move for 5 minutes to pump blood and lymph fluid through your body.

- **Walking and Aerobic Exercise.**

    According to Andrew Weil, walking is one of the best and safest forms of exercise -- not only because it is an exercise, but because the criss-cross swinging of the arms and legs and the counter-rotation of the pelvis and ribcage awaken "the electrical impulses" in your spine. Next time you walk, pay attention to how your right leg and left arm swing forward, while the ribcage very slightly rotates to the right and pelvis to the left. These body movements stimulate your brain, which affects your central nervous system. That's why insights, creative ideas and inspiration often come after a long walk. Walk daily! For your cardio endurance, walk 30 minutes to 1 hour at a brisk pace so that you are elevating your heart rate and your breathing deepens.

    > *Morning is the best time for aerobic exercise because it speeds the metabolism to burn twice as many calories throughout the day compared to the exercise done in the evening.*

- **Strengthen your pelvic floor.**

    The pelvic floor that supports our bladder, uterus and bowel weakens with age. To find your pelvic floor, try to stop the urine in mid flow. If you were able to do that, then you are contracting the right muscles. However, do not make it a practice of stopping the urinary flow as it actually can weaken the muscles and lead to urinary infections.

    Perform Kegel exercise to strengthen your pelvic floor muscles while seated, standing or driving. Contract your pelvic floor and hold for 5 seconds, gradually release contraction. Repeat 10 repetitions, 3 sets. Breathe naturally and make sure you avoid tucking your pelvis, tighten your thighs or buttocks. Pelvic floor muscles should be able to function in isolation.

- **Practice posture and emotional awareness.**

    Awareness: Slump in your chair and notice how this posture makes you feel. Now straighten yourself up and feel the difference in your outlook toward yourself and others.

    Throughout the day pay attention to how you are holding your head. Are you standing and sitting tall with feet grounded, lower back in neutral curves, abdominals toned, chest expanded, shoulders relaxed and head freely floating upwards or are you slumping while watching TV or sitting at the computer with your neck scrunched and shoulders tensed?

    In order to maintain a healthy aging body, we have to be aware of the inner energy system, so-called chakras. When our body is aligned and relaxed, our chakras in the spine are open and the energy flows through the body freely. The better our postural awareness throughout the day, the healthier we are. And vise versa, our chakras are affected by our emotional states. A heart chakra (energetic location) can close and chest collapse (physical location of the heart chakra) just by simply thinking a hurtful thought. The more we listen to our body and how it responds to our emotional states, the more we will be able to maintain the body-mind equilibrium and slow down the aging process.

In the beginning, it takes a lot of patience, self-correction and discipline to become aware of your posture. But eventually, it becomes easier; and you will need to think about it less often, because with practice your muscles will build a habitual memory. For instance, it will become easier for you to keep your abdominals engaged if throughout the day, you remind yourself to engage your core and check posture. Later it will become second nature to you and you will notice that with such "posture" comes a more positive outlook and greater self-confidence. Consider learning dance, martial arts, doing yoga or Pilates. These are all wonderful disciplines that teach you how to relate to yourself, others and objects in relation to you with grace, ease and awareness while the body is in movement.

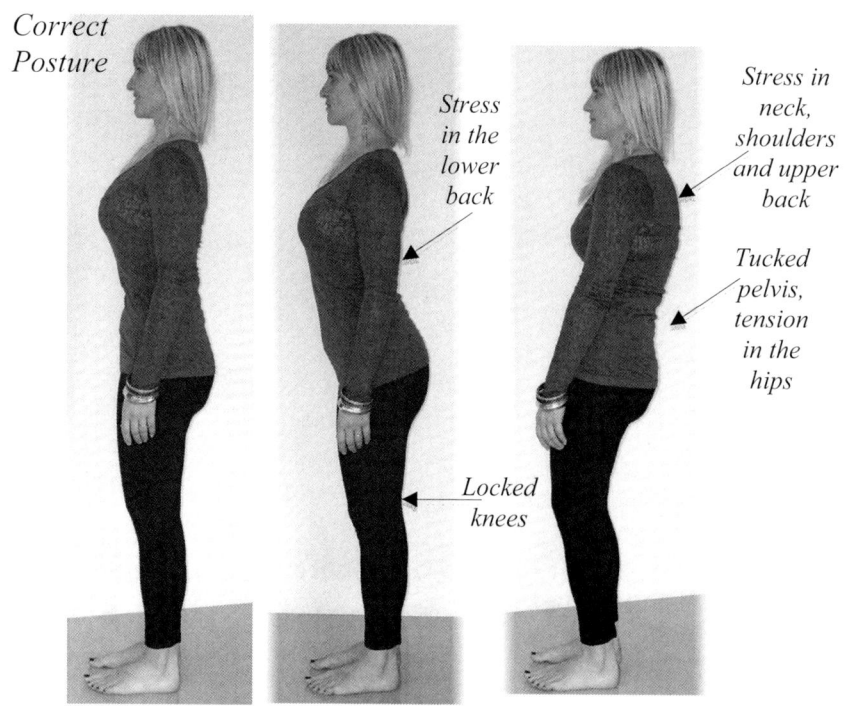

Sit with connection through your sitting bone, the bones in your buttocks. Keep lower back in neutral curves, abdominals toned, chest open, head floating up and feet grounded to the floor.

Correct

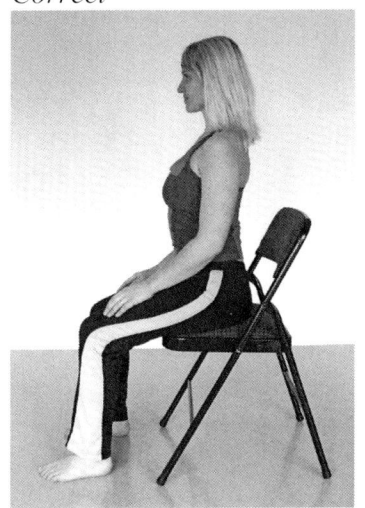

Correct

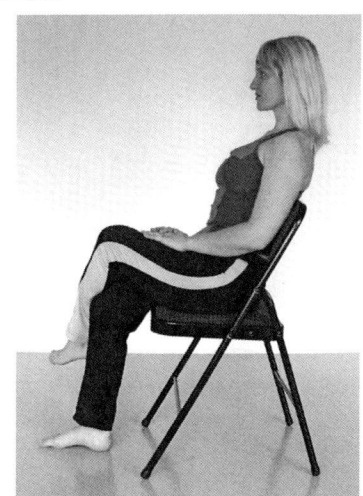

Incorrect

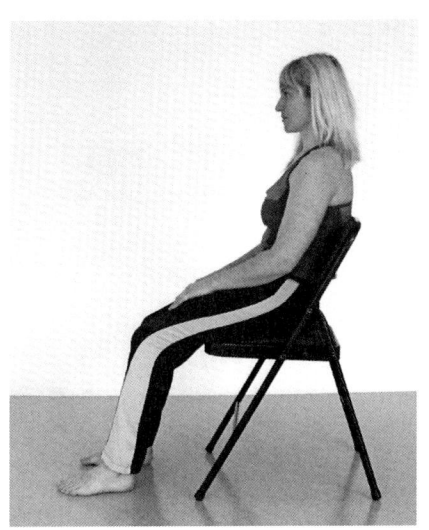

> Good posture requires good flexibility especially in your hip and lower back area. Notice that the cultures that do not use chairs develop healthy backs. I credit this to squatting they do as a regular daily life movement.

Face the object you are going to lift, stick you buttocks back, feel a deep crease at the front of your hips, keep your abdominals toned, shoulders stabilized, keeping object close to your body, use your leg muscles to pick and lift something.

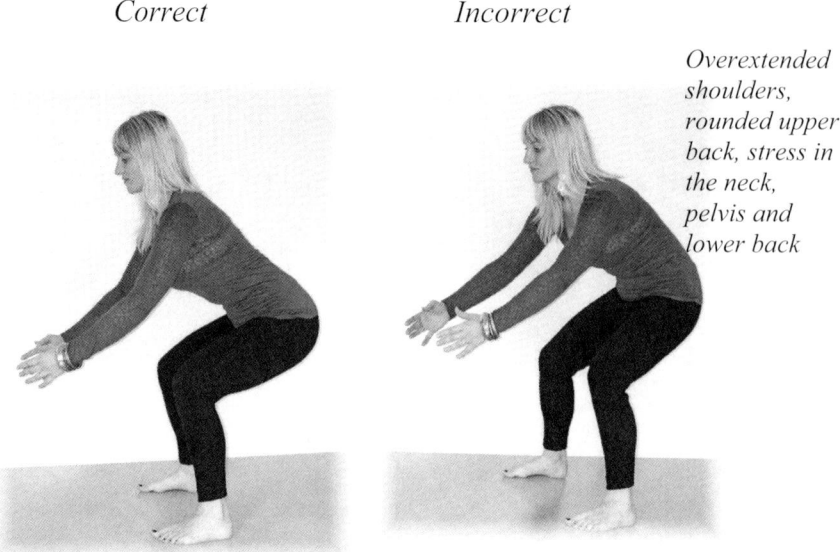

Correct *Incorrect*

Overextended shoulders, rounded upper back, stress in the neck, pelvis and lower back

Our body has been superbly engineered with its own shock absorbing system. By allowing the knees to be slightly bent in standing and moving, it is like having a cushioning system for the joints, including the spine.

Awareness: *Try this experiment! Stand with our feet hip distance apart and slightly bend your knees. Now move your hips and spine in different ways. Notice how it feels. Now try the same experiment but this time keep your knees straight. Have you noticed the difference? Yes, of course, when your knees are slightly bent your spine and hips have more mobility and freedom to move with grace and fluid movements without unnecessary tension and effort.*

♦ **Walk with spring in your feet!**

In times past, when there were no pavements and sidewalks, people climbed rocks, crossed river beds and walked across uneven terrains. With time our connection to the ground through our feet has been replaced by highly engineered footwear. Even though today's modern conveniences help us from stepping on the sharp objects and keep our feet warm, still the importance of moving barefoot and walking on uneven terrains often might be part of the solution in keeping your joints healthy.

Walking bare feet is very important as well. There are many proprioceptor nerves in the feet that tell us about our body positioning in space, teaching us about proper alignment. Also feet that are allowed to develop cushion our joints as we move.

Often we do not realize that the fascia, connective tissue in your feet, can be tight and restrict the normal gait. Use a tennis ball for this simple massage (for a deeper penetration use super ball) to release tight fascia. Stand on top of the ball and put the weight on it, hold for a second and repeat several times; move the ball to a new area and repeat massage on the whole sole of your foot. Make sure to include inner and outer edges of the feet. If your feet are tight, this massage might be painful; in that case, massage your feet seated and with less pressure.

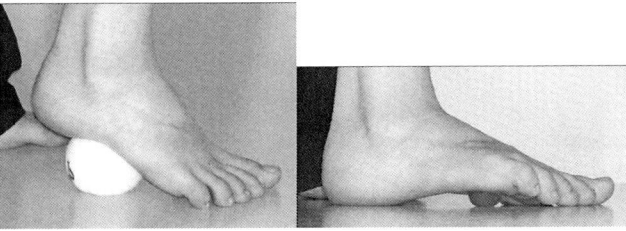

Walking Awareness: While walking, feel what is happening in your feet, pelvis, ribcage and shoulders. Feel a counter rotation: as your right leg swings forward, your pelvis rotates slightly to the left, simultaneously the left arm swings forward while the ribcage ever so slightly rotates to the right. Your right heel contacts the earth, roll through your whole foot and finally push off with the ball of the left foot to swing the left leg forward. The arms should swing freely at the shoulders and not at your elbows. Even worse, keeping your arms still and close to your body will require the body to move with unnecessary effort, creating tension in hips and shoulders. Keep your head up and aligned over your body, expand and radiate through your chest. Don't rush so fast that your head leads your body; don't be so slacking that your chest collapses and you keep looking under your feet. As you walk, gaze ahead while scanning surroundings about 30 feet ahead of you for any obstacles on the ground in the distance. Be aware of your surroundings!

- **Remember your hands and feet.**

There are many acupressure points on your hands and feet. Massage and hydrate your hands and feet daily. Pure oils and butters are the best moisturizers (almond oil, grape seed oil, hemp oil, coconut oil, shea butter). At least once a week, scrub your feet with a file to remove dead skin, then apply generous amounts of your favorite moisturizer and massage your feet. Put socks on and allow to soak in overnight.

> *Walk with your bare feet as often as possible to strengthen your ankles and feet muscles. Try walking on different surfaces like rocks, sand and grass. Stand on your tippy toes, walk backwards etc. The strongest and fastest running athletes are the ones that train barefoot.*

> *When working with your hands: washing dishes, weeding, cooking. Be aware of your whole palm, always do all your chores slowly and with*

> *awareness of your full contact to the object handling, with relaxed shoulders and gentle movement. Face your work and do not rush to get it finished. Try to make even your least enjoyable task as a meditative, learning experience. Do yourself a favor by living with Zen!*

- **Cold water therapy.**

Cold water tones your muscles, promotes circulation and metabolism. Splash your face with cool water in the morning to wake up your skin.

> *Cold water therapy is also excellent for aches and pains in your body!!! Athletes soak their body or a body part in tubs filled with ice. Cold water shower can work just as well. As my friend and naturopathic doctor, Jeannette, remarked: make sure you aim your shower head to your feet first, then your legs, moving upward. So, that you don't shock your heart and circulatory system.*
>
> *If you find it is too difficult to stand straight cold water, try alternating hot-cold, hot-cold, hot-cold. Always finish with cold water to close your pores, condition and tone your muscles.*
>
> *The cold water allowed to run down the back of your occipital area, the back of the neck, will help to ease the emotional tensions. This is the area where we carry our stress.*

- **Massage hemp oil on your body, especially joints.**

Hemp oil very closely matches our own skin's lipids. It is able to penetrate inside our cells and moisturize deeper layers of the skin; it also acts as a carrier of the healing properties of such anti-inflammatory herbs as arnica directly to the joints.

Here is how to perform self-massage using hemp oil. Start from your feet, then massage up your lower leg in the upward strokes toward your heart. When you reach your knee joints massage them in a circular motion. The oil will be absorbed through your skin, nourishing your skin and joints. Then move upward on your upper legs. Apply the oil in a circular motion on your hip joints. Continue up your belly, your chest, hands, forearms. In circular motions, massage elbows, up your upper arms and finish with a circular massage for your shoulder joints.

> *Aromatic Idea:*
> *Add a drop of invigorating peppermint or relaxing lavender essential oil to your massage.*

CONCLUSION

Remember that you are the creator of your life experience. Every day set your mind and heart on the intent to live life in such way that it will empower you to make wise choices. By your example radiate what it is like to live every moment of your life with enthusiasm and love.

Your heart beat, the pulse of the earth, the sound of the ocean, the breath, the silence of the night is a music to which we need to open our ears and listen more attentively, in time the lotus blossom opens up to turn every moment of our life into a dance of happiness. Dance every moment, dance very slowly and patiently, dance through your life like a child, see miracles everyday and be true to yourself! I wish that no matter how many times it seems difficult, rise up again, laugh often, reach for your dreams, take another step and live a life full of song, love and joy! Keep exploring your potential, inspire others and be inspired!

In India, Nepal and other Eastern countries, people greet and part by folding their hands in a prayer gesture at the heart and bowing to each other while saying "namaste." It means: I honor the place in me where there is light and goodness within, I honor the place in you where there is light and goodness, I honor a place in both of us, where there is only one of us. I was told by one of my students who visited Nepal that children who even have not learned to speak yet, when you greet them saying "namaste" they fold their hands in return. It is a beautiful way to relate to one another with respect and humility.

namaste

Bibliography

Bond, Mary. *The New Rules of Posture: How to Sit, Stand, and Move in the Modern World.* Rochester, VT: Healing Arts Press, 2007.

Bowman, Katy. "Movement as Medicine." *Natural Awakenings* February 2010: 12-13.

Buhner, Stephen Harrod. "The Secret Teachings of Plants." Rochester, VT: Bear & Company, 2004.

Chandler, Steve. *100 Ways to Motivate Yourself.* [Sound recording]. St. Paul, Minn.: HighBridge, 2000.

Clark, Nancy. *Nancy Clark's Sports Nutrition Guidebook.* Champaign, IL : Human Kinetics, 2009.

Cohen, Kenneth S. *The Way of Qigong = [Ch'i kung chi tao] : the Art and Science of Chinese Energy Healing.* New York : Ballantine Books, 1997.

Cohen, Kenneth S. *Honoring the Medicne.* New York : Random House, Inc., 2003.

Crowther, Ann, and Helena Petre. *Total Pilates: The Unique Step-by-Step Guide to Pilates at Home for Everybody.* London: Thorsons, 2003

"Epigenetics Diet, The." *IDEA Fitness Journal* July-August, 2011: 114.

Kurkland, Zack. *Morning Yoga Workouts.* Champaign, IL : Human Kinetics, 2007.

Lowe, Tamara. *Get Motivated!: Overcome Any Obstacle, Achieve Any Goal, and Accelerate Your Success with Motivational DNA.* New York: Doubleday, 2009.

McMillan, Sherri. "Shape Up with Sherri: Exercise, Fitness and Nutrition Tips to Help You Look and Feel Your Best." 2010. 12 Aug. <http://shapeupwithsherri.blogspot.com>.

Mogilner, Victoria. *Ancient Secrets of Facial Rejuvenation: a Non Surgical Approach to Youth and Well-Being.* Novato, Calif.: New World Library, 2006.

Price, Justin. "Understanding Muscles and Movement: From Theory to Practice." *IDEA Fitness Journal for ACE Certified Professionals* September 2010: 55-60.

Rodale. J. I. *My Own Technique of Eating for Health.* Emmaus, Penna.: Rodale Books, Inc., 1970.

Rosas, Debbie, and Carlos Rosas. *The Nia Technique: The High-Powered Energizing Workout that Gives You a New Body and a New Life.* New York: Broadway Books, 2004.

Trudeau, Kevin. *Natural Cures "They" Don't Want You to Know About.* Elk Grove Village, IL: Alliance Publishing Group, 2004.

Trudeau, Kevin. *Your Wish is Your Command. How to Manifest Your Desires.* [Sound recording].

Vennells, David F. *Reiki for Beginners: Mastering Natural Healing Techniques.* St. Paul, Minn.: Llewellyn Publications, 1999.

Weil, Andrew. *Spontaneous Healing: How to Discover and Enhance Your Body's Natural Ability to Maintain and Heal Itself.* Hampton Falls, N.H.: Beeker Large Print, 1995.

Wharton, Jim, and Phil Wharton. *The Wharton's Back Book: End Back Pain – Now And Forever - with This Simple, Revolutionary Program.* Emmaus, Pennsylvania: Rodale, 2003.

About Author

Violeta Bailets is a fitness and wellness professional, helping people to feel their best since 1994 through movement, coaching, inspiration and writings. Creator of the YoChi™ Dance, YoChi™ Walk and YoChi™ Core– fitness programs that fuse yoga, Pilates, dance and walking outdoors with chi gong.

Your comments are very welcome, write to:

Violeta Bailets

131 Oakwood Dr.

St. Helens, OR 97051

USA

503- 914-9693

violeta@bodymotionstudio.biz

www.bodymotionstudio.biz

Special Offer: write a review of the book and receive
5 minute Facial Acupressure and Exercise Booklet

The exercises tone muscles and promote blood flow; the increased blood flow stimulates the formation of collagen, making the skin more pliable. Oriental acupressure and massage techniques release tension, promote removal of toxic waste from under the skin. Relieve headaches and unblock energy in the face, neck and head.